OSMOSIS

ELECTROCARDIOGRAPHY ESSENTIALS

Edition: 1.02

Fergus Baird, MA
Charles B. Davis, BS
Lyndsay Day, MA
Rishi Desai, MD, MPH
Tanner Marshall, MS
Kyle Slinn, RN, MEd

2017

We'd like to thank our Osmosis Prime members, our supporters, the hundreds of volunteers who double check our facts and translate our videos, and of course, our viewers on YouTube and Wikipedia. You all have played a huge part in helping us make the best learning experiences possible.

If you find any mistakes, let us know here:
https://goo.gl/forms/DjaI70T3Iicqckpi1

Osmosis Team

Hillary Acer, BA
John Bafford, BS
Fergus Baird, MA
Sarah Clifford, BMBS, BS
Andrea Day, MA
Harry Delaney, MBChB
Rishi Desai, MD, MPH
Evan Debevec-McKenney, BA
Allison Dollar, BFA

Caleb Furnas, MA
Shiv Gaglani, MBA
Sam Gillespie, BSc
Ryan Haynes, PhD
Heidi Hildebrandt, MA
Thasin Jaigirdar, BA
Justin Ling, MD
Tanner Marshall, MS
Sam Miller, BA
Brandon Newton, BBA,
Brittany Norton, MFA

Viviana Popa, MD candidate
Vishal Punwani, MD
Kyle Slinn, RN, MEd
Diana Stanley, MBA
Sean Tackett, MD, MPH
Ashley Thompson, BSc
Marisa Pedron, BA
Vincent Waldman, PhD
Yifan Xiao, MD

AUTHORS

Fergus Baird is a copywriter, editor and textbook designer at Osmosis, and dabbles in a little scriptwriting for the YouTube channel and textbooks as well.

Before moving to Canada, Fergus lived in a small village in Scotland. He earned his Master's degree in English literature at Concordia University in Montréal, writing his thesis on history and the graphic novel. Before joining Team Osmosis, Fergus worked as a gif curator, a movie subtitler, a meme master and a ghost writer, and spent a year teaching elementary school kids in Japan.

When he's not eating or cooking elaborate meals for his friends, Fergus spends his spare time playing video games and the theremin, drawing strange pictures, and consuming horror media in all its gruesome forms.

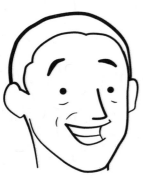

Fergus Baird
MA

Rishi is a pediatric infectious disease physician at Stanford University and serves as the Chief Medical Officer at Osmosis. He recently led the Khan Academy Medicine team, which put together a collection of videos and questions for students entering the health sciences.

With the help of his parents and teachers, Rishi completed high school and received his BS in Microbiology from UCLA by the age of 18. He completed his medical training at UCSF, pediatric residency at Boston Children's Hospital, and did an infectious disease fellowship at Children's Hospital Los Angeles. He earned his MPH in epidemiology at UCLA, and then spent two years chasing down infectious disease outbreaks for the Centers for Disease Control and Prevention, before beginning his work in online medical education.

In his spare time, Rishi enjoys watching his son torment the family dog, while eating nature's finest fruit—the raspberry!

Rishi Desai
MD, MPH

Tanner's the voice and illustrator behind the majority of Osmosis videos (as well as a few icons, graphics, and cartoons scattered around Osmosis). Tanner got both his undergrad and graduate degree in biomedical engineering from the University of Wisconsin-Madison (Go Badgers!), before moving out to Portland, OR and starting his engineering career.

After working in the cardiac rhythm management business for bit, he stumbled upon the two goofballs Rishi and Kyle, and began working alongside (well, technically under, but who's counting!) them producing openly accessible videos for Khan Academy Medicine.

In addition to being an enthusiast for science education and being halfway-decent with a drawing tablet, he also takes pride in his diverse collection of hats (including both beanies and baseball caps), his skills on the ultimate frisbee field, and his vast knowledge of the *Star Wars* universe.

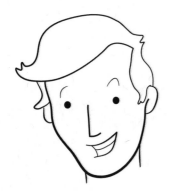

Tanner Marshall
MS

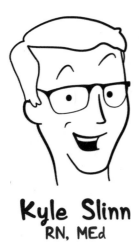

Kyle Slinn
RN, MEd

Kyle is a project manager and instructional designer at Osmosis. He wears many hats, managing volunteers and contractors, designing future projects, producing videos, leading internationalization efforts, and designing Osmosis's textbooks. A jack-of-all-trades. Before Osmosis he worked as a project coordinator for Khan Academy Medicine where he managed the creation of videos, questions, and text-based articles for MCAT and NCLEX-RN students.

Kyle also worked in the pediatric intensive care unit as a nurse at the Children's Hospital of Eastern Ontario, in Ottawa, Canada. He received his Bachelors of Science in Nursing from the University of Ottawa and holds a Masters of Education in Distance Education from Athabasca University.

With his free time Kyle loves to go on adventures, hang out with friends, play board games, bake bread, and play musical instruments.

ASSOCIATED AUTHORS

Charles B. Davis
BS

Charlie writes content for Osmosis. He completed his BS in Biochemistry, Cell and Molecular Biology at Drake University. Next, he started a band and moved to New York City where he spent his days above ground as a research technician at Memorial Sloan Kettering Cancer Center, and his nights playing piano and ukulele in unfinished basements of Queens. He is currently a fourth-year medical student at the University of Kansas School of Medicine and will pursue a residency in radiology.

Charlie believes that people are naturally curious and that it's the responsibility of educators to cultivate that curiosity with entertaining content presentations. In his free time, Charlie enjoys eating, reading science fiction, and performing random acts of kindness.

Lyndsay Day
MA

Lyndsay copyedits for Osmosis. This means she helps scriptwriters convey meaning and tone through grammar, and she helps clarify content. Her favourite punctuation mark is the semicolon; the Oxford comma is a close second. As a teaching assistant, Lyndsay enjoys encouraging students to develop their own individual writing "voices." She is also working on a PhD in English Literature.

Lyndsay has enjoyed using her research and writing skills in new contexts while working for Osmosis. Reading scripts on a variety of topics has also given her a greater appreciation of how hard our bodies work to stay healthy.

In her free time, Lyndsay enjoys snuggling cats (particularly her sister Andrea's cat, Mortimer), doing crafts, and reading comic books.

REVIEWERS

Creating accurate content is really hard. Thousands of eyeballs will look at our work for years to come and inevitably we'll have missed something, or something will go out of date. What's nice about our way of producing content is we get a lot of feedback really fast. Within 24 hours of releasing a video we've meticulously crafted and reviewed, we get thousands of views. In the rare instance there's a mistake, our audience is always quick to use the comment feature to point out where we went wrong. Yep, we're listening! We read every single comment across all of our videos. Whenever someone points out a factual inaccuracy, we update our video and rerelease it. Currently, YouTube doesn't allow editions of videos to exist. When we rerelease a video, we're effectively pulling the existing, well-established and easily searchable video out of circulation and putting a new, less searchable video in its place. There have been several times where our team has silently cried inside as we take down our most viewed video in the name of scientific accuracy. In the end, though, the result is that we can confidently say our videos (and textbooks) are factually accurate.

We'd like to thank the following people who have given us so much guidance as we've created our content.

Adeeb Aghdassi, MD	**Lisa Miklush**, PhD, RNC, CNS
Jodi Berndt, PhD	**Kevin F. Moynahan**, MD
John Bloom, MD	**Nacole T. Riccaboni**, BSN, RN, CCRN-CMC
Armando Hasudungan Faigl, BBiomedSc	**Thomas M. Schmid**, PhD
Jennifer French, MEd	**Kathy W. Smith**, MD
Vanita Gaglani, RPT	**Eric Strong**, MD
Kristine Krafts, MD	**Todd W. Vanderah**, PhD

FOREWORD

We're excited to introduce you to *Osmosis Electrocardiography Essentials*, the second title in our textbook series. We founded Osmosis as medical students at Johns Hopkins, back when only 118 of our classmates were using the platform. Fast forward a few years and the Osmosis audience has grown to more than 350,000 medical & health science students internationally. Our team now includes over two dozen incredibly intelligent and passionate people who work hard to provide you the best education so that, ultimately, you can provide your future patients with the best care possible. We're proud of the work that the Osmosis content team has done to fulfill this mission, with this book being the latest step on that path.

Being able to read an electrocardiogram is an essential skill for any medical doctor. Having a healthy heart means having a healthy heartbeat, and the best way to evaluate that is by looking at an ECG. We've designed this book to be a quick primer on the essentials of electrocardiography. By the time you've finished these 8 short chapters, you'll be familiar with the fundamentals of electrocardiography, and will be able to easily recognize the difference between a healthy QRS complex and an abnormal one, so that you can spot life-threatening conditions like ventricular fibrillation and myocardial ischemia.

While you may not be able to sleep with your head on this textbook and "learn by Osmosis," you can use the powerful & comprehensive Osmosis learning platform to watch our electrocardiography videos and actively quiz yourself with tens of thousands of associated multiple choice questions & flashcards. We encourage you to visit www.osmosis.org to learn more.

Best of luck Osmosing!

Shiv Gaglani
MBA
Co-founder & CEO

Ryan Haynes
PhD
Co-founder & CTO

Watch our new videos every week:
www.youtube.com/osmosis

Follow us on Facebook:
www.facebook.com/osmoseit

Follow us on Twitter:
@osmoseit

Follow us on Instagram:
@osmosismed

Check out our other content!
www.osmosis.org

Join our growing community on Reddit:
www.reddit.com/r/osmoseit

CONTENTS

READ OUR OTHER BOOKS!

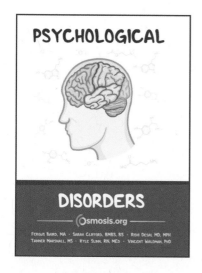

OSMOSIS PSYCHOLOGICAL DISORDERS

Experience Osmosis' mental health videos in book form! *Osmosis Psychological Disorders* covers over 30 topics on everything from ADHD and autism to opioid use dependence, with clear, concise descriptions, 350+ full-color illustrations and extra wide margins for notes. Don't study it, Osmose it!

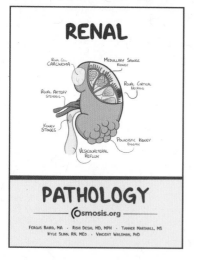

OSMOSIS RENAL PATHOLOGY

Experience Osmosis' renal pathology videos in book form! *Osmosis Renal Pathology* covers over 50 topics on everything from acute pyelonephritis to renal tubular acidosis, with clear, concise descriptions, over 580 full-color illustrations and extra wide margins for notes. Don't study it, Osmose it!

BUY THESE AND MORE AT

shop.osmosis.org

Electrocardiography Basics

TAKE NOTES **HERE!**

osmosis.org/learn/ecg_basics

An electrocardiogram is also known as an ECG; the Dutch and German version of the word, *elektrokardiogram*, is shortened to EKG. It is a tool used to visualize, or "gram," the electricity, or "electro," that flows through the heart, or "cardio." Specifically, a 12-lead ECG tracing shows how the depolarization wave, which is a wave of positive charge, moves during each heartbeat, by providing the perspectives of different sets of electrodes. This particular set of electrodes is called lead II; one electrode is placed on the right arm and the other on the left leg. Essentially, when the wave's moving toward the left leg electrode, you get a positive deflection. This big, positive deflection corresponds to the wave moving down the septum **(Figure 1.1)**.

To understand the basics, let's start with an example of how we can look at the heart with only one pair of electrodes: a positive and a negative one **(Figure 1.2; Figure 1.3)**. These electrodes detect the charge on the *outside* of the cell.

Remember, at rest, cells are negatively charged relative to the slightly positive outside environment; let's make these cells red **(Figure 1.4)**. When they depolarize, the cells become positively charged, leaving a slightly negative charge in the outside environment; let's make these green **(Figure 1.5)**. If we freeze this "wave of depolarization" as it's moving through the cells, half the cells are negative, or depolarized, and half are positive and resting, so there's a difference in charge across this set of cells **(Figure 1.6)**. You can think of the charge difference as a *dipole*, because there are two electrical poles. We can draw this dipole out as an arrow, or vector, pointing towards the positive charge **(Figure 1.7)**. The electrodes detect charge on the *outside* of the cell, so this points toward where the positive charge is, outside **(Figure 1.8)**.

Figure 1.1

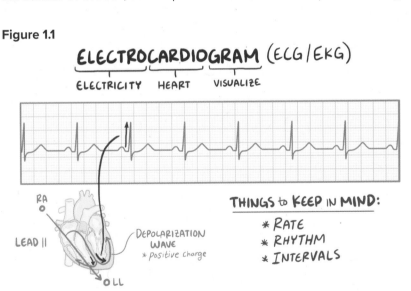

Figure 1.2   **Figure 1.3**

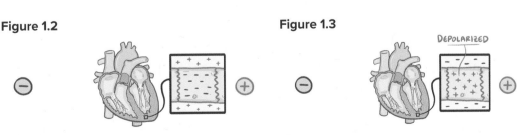

Figure 1.4

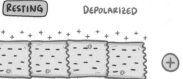

Figure 1.5

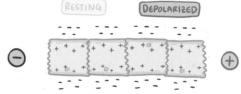

Figure 1.6

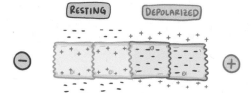

Figure 1.7

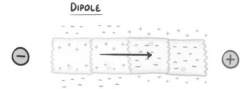

Figure 1.8

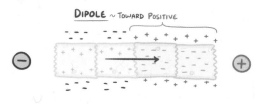

Figure 1.9

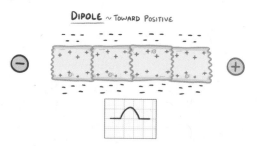

Figure 1.10

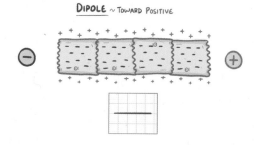

Figure 1.11

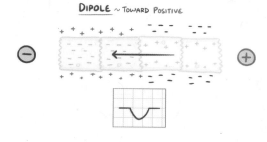

Figure 1.12

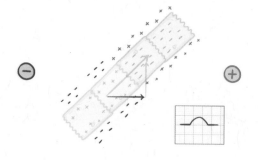

Figure 1.13

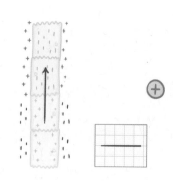

DEPOLARIZATION & DIPOLE VECTORS

Now, if there's a dipole vector pointing toward the positive electrode, then the ECG tracing shows it as a positive deflection; the bigger the dipole, the bigger the deflection **(Figure 1.9)**. If we unpause this, then everything becomes depolarized. Since there's no *difference in charge*, there's no dipole, and thus no deflection **(Figure 1.10)**. Moments later a wave of *repolarization* goes through and the cells become negative once again. Pausing halfway through again, now the dipole vector goes in the opposite direction and faces the negative electrode; this means that there will be a negative ECG tracing **(Figure 1.11)**. Again, the bigger the dipole is, the bigger the negative deflection is.

Even though it'd be nice if the depolarization wave lined up perfectly with the electrodes, usually that's not the case. So, we simply look at the vector component parallel to that electrode. For example, let's say the depolarization happened this way, at an angle; then, we'd simply break the vector into two parts **(Figure 1.12)**. The one we care about is going towards the positive electrode, which causes a deflection, even though it's a slightly smaller deflection than previously. In other words, the size of the deflection on the ECG tracing always corresponds to the magnitude, or size, of the dipole in the direction of the electrode. The perpendicular component isn't pointing at the electrodes, so it doesn't cause any deflection. In fact, if there's a depolarization wave that goes straight up, perpendicular to the positive and negative electrodes, there would be no deflection **(Figure 1.13)**!

LIMB & CHEST LEADS

In a standard ECG, there are 10 electrodes: four limb electrodes, with one each on the left arm, right arm, left leg, and right leg; and six precordial electrodes, V_1 through V_6, that wrap around the chest. The right leg electrode is usually used as a neutral lead. The heart is a three-dimensional organ, so V_1 through V_6 line up in the transverse, or horizontal, plane of the heart. Each electrode is set up to detect any wave of positive charge coming towards it. These are collectively called the chest leads **(Figure 1.14)**.

Figure 1.14

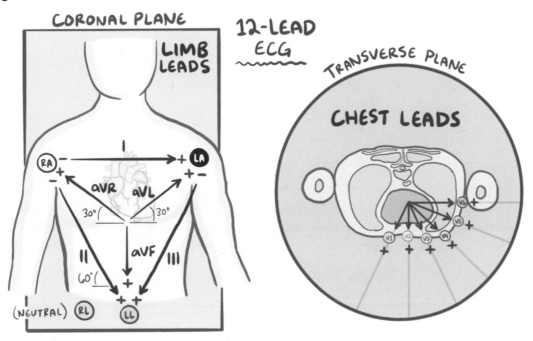

Figure 1.15

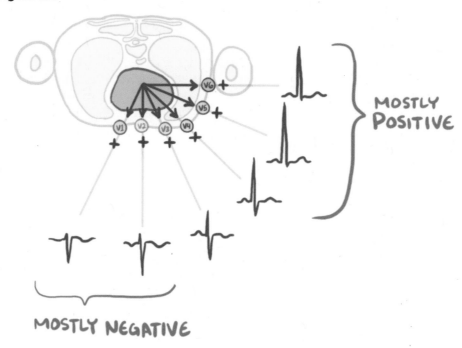

MOSTLY POSITIVE

MOSTLY NEGATIVE

Figure 1.16

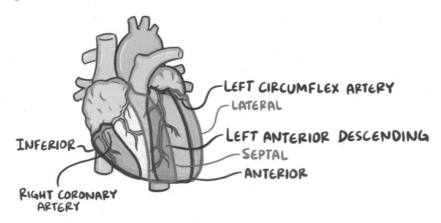

LEFT CIRCUMFLEX ARTERY
LATERAL
LEFT ANTERIOR DESCENDING
SEPTAL
ANTERIOR
INFERIOR
RIGHT CORONARY ARTERY

Figure 1.17

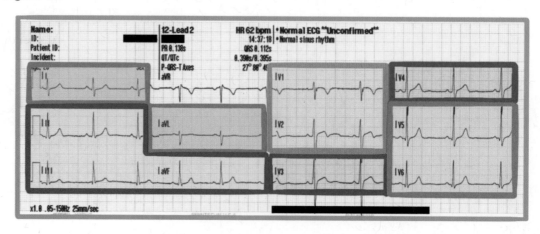

Meanwhile, in the coronal plane, the non-neutral leads are called augmented vector right, or aVR, on the right arm, and augmented vector left, or aVL, on the left arm. Both of these leads are represented as vectors that are 30 degrees up from the horizontal line. Augmented vector foot, or aVF, is on the left foot, which anatomically isn't straight down, but it's close enough that it ends up representing the vector facing straight down on the diagram. Just like the precordial electrodes, aVR, aVL, and aVF detect any positive deflection coming towards them. Now, in addition to these three limb leads, there are also bipolar limb leads called lead I, lead II, and lead III, which are recorded using two electrodes instead of just one. Lead I uses the RA as the negative pole and LA as the positive pole, forming a vector that goes to the right. Lead II uses aVR as the negative pole and aVF as the positive pole, forming a vector that goes to the +60 degree mark. Finally, lead III uses aVL as the negative pole and aVF as the positive pole, forming a vector that goes to the +120 degree mark. So, in total you've got six leads from the limb leads and six from the chest leads, which add up to 12 leads total; in other words, you have a 12-lead ECG.

THE VALUE OF DIFFERENT VIEWPOINTS

Having different views of the heart is important, because they make it possible for you to see how the wave of depolarization moves through the heart according to each viewpoint. For example, consider how the six chest leads, V_1 through V_6, register the depolarization wave form called the QRS complex. The very same depolarization wave might appear mostly negative in V_1 and V_2, isoelectric in V_3, and mostly positive in V_4, V_5, and V_6, because the exact direction and magnitude of the vectors are at different points in time . Similarly, each of the frontal plane leads produces its own perspective of the depolarization wave **(Figure 1.15)**.

The limb leads and chest leads can be grouped based on the regions of the heart that they are nearest, as we've indicated in this color-coded chart **(Figure 1.16; Figure 1.17)**. Problems in specific leads, or groups of leads, suggests that there may be a specific region of the heart affected by a disease. Leads II, III, and aVF are "inferior" leads because they're near the inferior wall of the heart, which receives blood from the right coronary artery. Leads I and aVL, along with two of the chest leads, V_5 and V_6, are considered "lateral" leads because they're near the lateral wall of the heart, which receives blood from the left circumflex artery. Finally, V_1 and V_2 are considered "septal" leads because they're nearest to the interventricular septum, and V_3 and V_4 are "anterior" leads because they're nearest the anterior wall of the heart. Both of the septal and anterior regions are served by the left anterior descending artery.

Figure 1.18

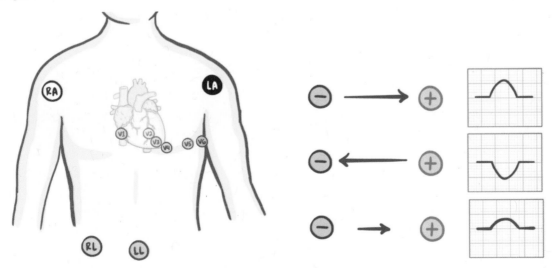

SUMMARY

All right, let's quickly recap. In a standard ECG there are 10 electrodes: four limb electrodes and six precordial electrodes that wrap around the chest. These electrodes are used to make 12 leads, each of which illustrates the movement of positive charge on the outside of heart cells. The ECG tracing shows a depolarization wave moving towards an electrode as a positive deflection, and one moving away as a negative deflection; each is proportional to the size of the dipole. The benefit of being able to see different views of the heart is that it makes it easier to see how the wave of depolarization moves, which provides valuable information about the heart's structure and function **(Figure 1.18; Figure 1.19)**.

Figure 1.19

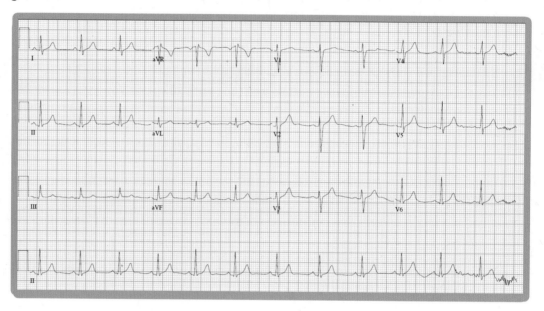

Normal Sinus Rhythm

osmosis.org/learn/normal_sinus_rhythm

To read an ECG, it's important to first understand what a normal sinus rhythm looks like **(Figure 2.1)**. To do that, let's look at a single heartbeat on an ECG from the viewpoint of lead II.

DEPOLARIZATION

In a healthy heart, everything starts at the sinoatrial node, or SA node, which is a little patch of tissue in the wall of the right atrium full of pacemaker cells. When one of these pacemaker cells depolarizes, a wave of positive charge spreads outward; overall, it moves from the SA node towards the apex of the heart, so it aligns nicely with the lead II vector **(Figure 2.2)**.

Figure 2.1

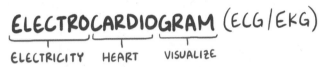

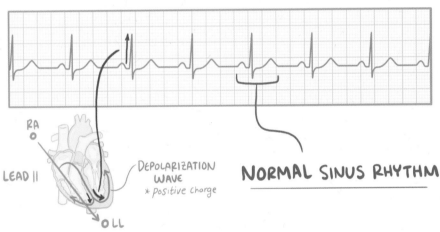

Figure 2.2

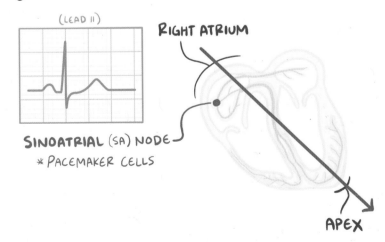

Figure 2.3

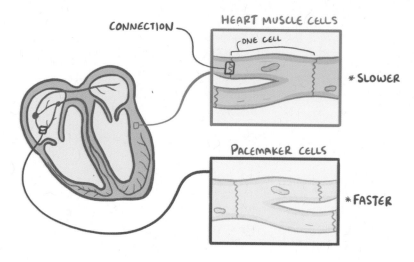

Figure 2.4

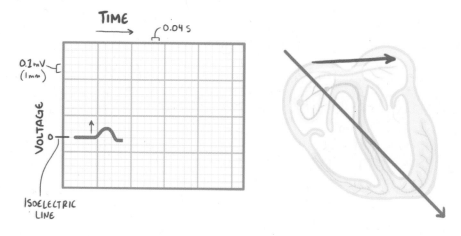

Figure 2.5

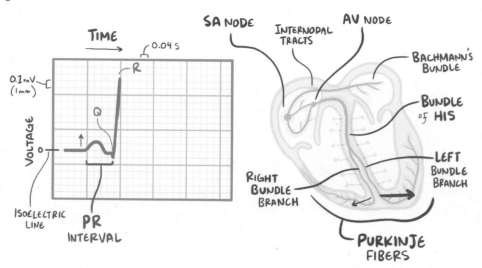

Now, the heart muscle cells are often described as having a functional syncytium because even though each one cell has its own cell membrane, the cells also have tiny connections, or openings, between them. That means that during a depolarization wave ions can flow right from one cell to the next. It's also important to note that the depolarization wave moves at two different speeds through the heart. In the pacemaker cells, which are special types of cardiomyocytes laid out like highways through the heart, it moves really fast. It moves more slowly through the rest of myocytes that do the contracting; the depolarization wave moves through these cells like a car travelling through small, congested streets **(Figure 2.3)**.

READING DEPOLARIZATION ON AN ECG

The ECG measures out changes in time on the X-axis, where one small box is 0.04 s, and voltage on the Y-axis, with each small box equal to 0.1 mV, which is sometimes called 1 mm voltage. Zero is called the "isoelectric line." Every time there's positive voltage, there's an upward deflection *above* the isoelectric line, and every time there's negative voltage, there's a downward deflection *below* the isoelectric line. So, a depolarization wave starts in the SA node, then goes through *atrial intranodal tracts*, which is also called Bachmann's bundle, and travels over to the left atrium so that both atria basically depolarize together. The overall direction of that depolarization wave is in the same direction as the lead II vector, so that's considered positive voltage, and there's a positive deflection called the P wave **(Figure 2.4)**.

Meanwhile, the signal also gets carried from the SA node to the atrioventricular node, or AV node; here, it gets delayed for a bit, which allows the atria to fully contract and fill the ventricles with blood. During this delay, there is no depolarization wave moving towards or away from lead II, so this appears as a flat line. The interval from the beginning of the P wave through this flat portion is called the PR interval. From there, the signal goes through the pacemaker cells that make up the bundle of His, and into the left bundle branch and right bundle branches. In addition to moving through the fast pacemaker cells, the signal also travels through the slow myocytes in the interventricular septum; this direction is slightly away from the lead II vector, because there is a lot of this tissue. This creates a tiny negative deflection on the ECG: a Q wave **(Figure 2.5)**.

From there, the depolarization wave flows down into the Purkinje fibers. Since the largest vectors are the ones in the left ventricle, this is in the direction of lead II; this creates a large positive deflection on the ECG: an R wave. The apex of the heart depolarizes first, but then the wave moves back up to depolarize the top of the ventricles, which is in a direction away from lead II; this causes a slight negative deflection on the ECG: an S wave. Together, ventricular depolarization creates what is called the QRS complex **(Figure 2.6)**.

Figure 2.6

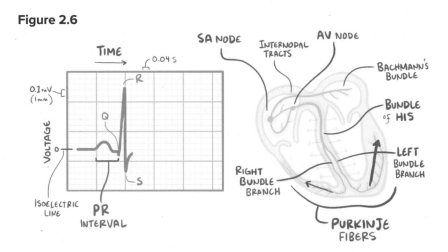

Figure 2.7

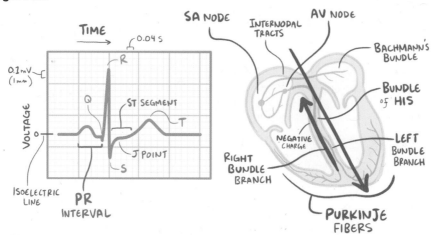

After tissue depolarizes, there is a brief period of time when there is no change in electrical activity; thus, the ECG goes back to the isoelectric line. The exact point at which it hits that line is called the J point. For a brief time, there is no net change in electrical activity; this is the ST segment. After that, the ventricles have to repolarize or become negative once more in order to reset themselves in preparation for another wave of depolarization.

Now, *repolarization* moves in an overall direction upward, opposite the direction of lead II. You might think that it should be a negative deflection, but really it's a *positive* deflection, because this time it's a wave of *negative* charge; essentially, now when it's moving opposite to lead II, it's a positive deflection on ECG. This final wave is called the T wave **(Figure 2.7)**.

The T wave is more spread out over time than the QRS complex because repolarization is a slower process that takes place at slightly different times for each cardiomyocyte, instead of happening all at once, as with depolarization. It's also worth mentioning that atrial repolarization doesn't usually show up at all on the ECG because the small vectors it creates get lost in much larger vectors created by the the QRS complex.

SUMMARY

All right, let's quickly recap. On an ECG, there's a P wave, which corresponds to the atrial depolarization wave, followed by an isoelectric line, when the depolarization wave goes through the AV node. After that, there's a QRS complex, which represents ventricular depolarization, followed by another brief isoelectric pause, called the ST segment. Finally, there's a T wave, which represents ventricular repolarization **(Figure 2.8)**.

Figure 2.8

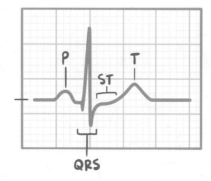
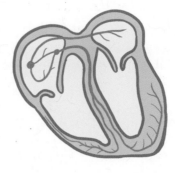

Rate & Rhythm

osmosis.org/learn/ecg_rate_and_rhythm

To read an ECG, there are a few key elements to keep in mind; one is to figure out the rate and rhythm **(Figure 3.1)**. There are a couple of ways to figure out the heart rate on an ECG.

THE BOX METHOD

The first is called the "box method," because you count the number of boxes between heartbeats. Each small box represents 0.04 seconds, and each big box is made up of five small boxes, so each big box is 0.2 seconds. To use this method, you count the number of small boxes between R waves, because R waves are tall, pointy, and easy to see in lead II of an ECG strip. You can find an R wave that has a peak that falls at the beginning of a box, and then count up how many boxes until the same point on the next R wave. Let's say that there are four big boxes and one and a half small boxes between two R waves. In other words, there are 4 x 5 + 1.5 = 21.5 small boxes. This means that there's 0.04 seconds x 21.5, or .86 seconds, between heartbeats. Now, to get a result that's a little more meaningful, we can take the inverse, which is one over 0.86 beats per second, or 1.16 beats per second. Now, there are 60 seconds in a minute, so if we multiply that by 60, we end up with 70 beats per minute—the heart rate **(Figure 3.2)**!

Now, if the distance between two R waves is exactly one big box, then the heart rate would be 300 beats per minute, which is *really* fast. If R waves are two big boxes apart, or 0.4 seconds apart, then the heart rate is 150 beats per minute. Three big boxes apart is 100 beats per minute, and four, five, and six big boxes apart is 75, 60, and 50 beats per minute respectively. Remembering these numbers makes it easier to make a rough estimate. For example, if there are three to four large boxes between R waves, then the heart rate must be between 75 and 100 beats per minute **(Figure 3.3)**.

Figure 3.1

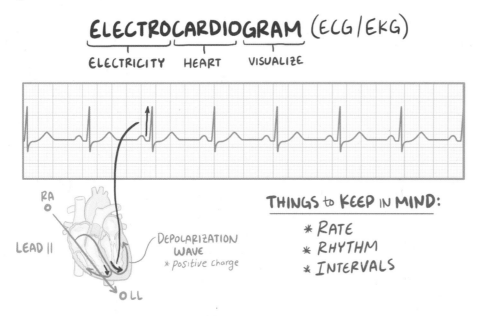

ELECTROCARDIOGRAM (ECG/EKG)

ELECTRICITY   HEART   VISUALIZE

RA

LEAD II

DEPOLARIZATION WAVE
* positive charge

O LL

THINGS to KEEP IN MIND:
* RATE
* RHYTHM
* INTERVALS

Figure 3.2

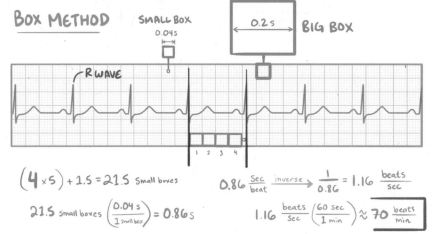

BOX METHOD

SMALL BOX
0.04s

0.2s — BIG BOX

R WAVE

1 2 3 4

$(4 \times 5) + 1.5 = 21.5$ small boxes

$21.5 \text{ small boxes} \left(\frac{0.04 \text{ s}}{1 \text{ small box}} \right) = 0.86 \text{ s}$

$0.86 \frac{\text{sec}}{\text{beat}} \xrightarrow{\text{inverse}} \frac{1}{0.86} = 1.16 \frac{\text{beats}}{\text{sec}}$

$1.16 \frac{\text{beats}}{\text{sec}} \left(\frac{60 \text{ sec}}{1 \text{ min}} \right) \approx 70 \frac{\text{beats}}{\text{min}}$

Figure 3.3

BOX METHOD

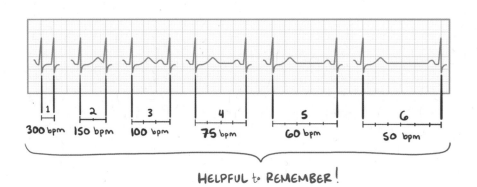

1 — 300 bpm
2 — 150 bpm
3 — 100 bpm
4 — 75 bpm
5 — 60 bpm
6 — 50 bpm

HELPFUL to REMEMBER!

Figure 3.4

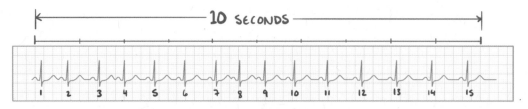

10 SECONDS

1 2 3 4 5 6 7 8 9 10 11 12 13 14 15

$15 \times 6 = 90 \text{ bpm}$

$\frac{15 \text{ beats}}{10 \text{ seconds}} \left(\frac{60 \text{ seconds}}{1 \text{ minute}} \right) = 15 \text{ beats} \left(\frac{6}{\text{min}} \right) = 90 \frac{\text{beats}}{\text{min}}$

Figure 3.5

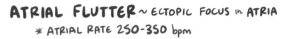

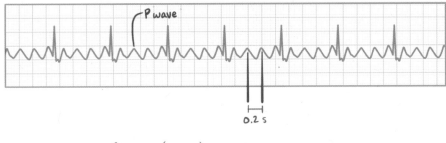

NUMBER OF BEATS PER TEN SECONDS

Counting the number of beats in ten seconds, the standard length of time on the rhythm strip portion of a 12-lead ECG is another method you can use to determine heart rate. In this case, we've got 15 beats. All you need to do is multiply this by six to get the heart rate, which would be 90 beats per minute. The reason this little trick works is that you've got 15 beats per 10 seconds, and again, to convert to *per minute* you multiply by 60 seconds in a minute. Looking at this, we see that 60 / 10 = 6 per minute. So, 6 x 15 = 90 beats per minute **(Figure 3.4)**.

IRREGULAR HEART RATES AND RHYTHMS

If the heart rate is too slow or too fast, it could be because something other than the SA node is pacing the heart rate. For example, there could be atrial flutter, which is when an ectopic focus in the atria, such as an irritated atrial cell, starts to spontaneously fire between 250-350 depolarizations per minute; then, only one out of every few atrial depolarizations passes through to the ventricles.

To calculate the atrial rate, you can use the same method as before, except you look at P waves instead of R waves. If one P wave begins on a heavy line, and the next P wave begins on the next heavy line, or 0.2 seconds later, then again, you've got one beat for every 0.2 seconds; multiplying by the 60 seconds in a minute, you get 300 beats per minute. You could also remember that one big box is equal to 300 bpm **(Figure 3.5)**.

Another situation is atrial fibrillation, which is when there are multiple ectopic foci in the atria that start firing all at once; the atrial rate can increase to 350-450 beats per minute. In this situation, only the occasional firing of an ectopic focus that happens to be near the AV node is able to make it through and down to the ventricles. The ectopic foci fire too quickly for the atria to be fully depolarized by any one of them, so there are few, if any, actual P waves. So, without P waves, there's not a reliable method of determining the atrial rate just by looking at the ECG strip. Also, the heart rate is really just an estimate, because at this point the heart is just quivering **(Figure 3.6)**.

Normally on an ECG, one waveform's P wave, QRS complex, and T wave look just like the next one's, almost like they were copied and pasted one right after another. That's how a regular rhythm looks; the heart moves like a smooth dancer on rhythm. An irregular rhythm, on the other hand, is when there's any change in the appearance, sequence, or timing of these waves **(Figure 3.7)**.

Figure 3.6

ATRIAL FIBRILLATION ~ MULTIPLE ECTOPIC FOCI
* ATRIAL RATE 350-450 bpm

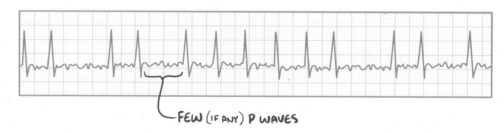

└─ FEW (IF ANY) P WAVES

* **NO** RELIABLE WAY to READ ATRIAL RATE
  └─ ATRIA QUIVERING

Figure 3.7

* REGULAR RHYTHM *

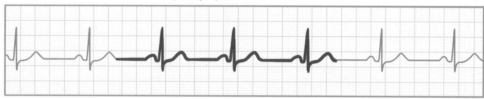

* IRREGULAR RHYTHM *

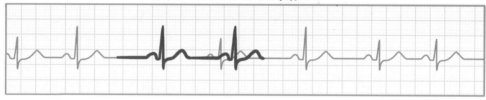

~ ANY CHANGE in APPEARANCE, SEQUENCE, or TIMING ~

Figure 3.8

* IRREGULAR RHYTHM *

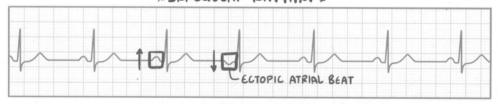

└─ ECTOPIC ATRIAL BEAT

* DOES EVERY PART **LOOK** the SAME?
  └─ P WAVE?
  └─ QRS COMPLEX?
  └─ T WAVE?

Figure 3.9

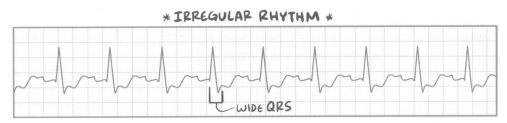

Figure 3.10

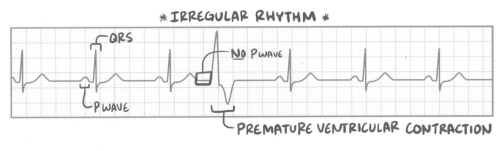

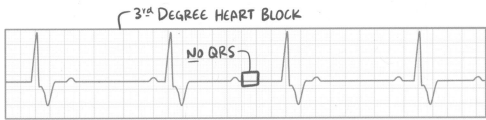

To help identify an irregular rhythm, it helps to ask if every part of the waveform, including the P wave, QRS complex, and T wave, looks exactly the same as the others. If not, it could mean that there's an ectopic beat, which means that it may have originated from an abnormal spot in the atria or ventricles. For example, this first P wave is deflected upwards and the second is deflected downward, which indicates that it's an ectopic beat **(Figure 3.8)**.

Alternatively, an odd-looking waveform may have originated from the normal spot, the sinoatrial node, but was thrown off course; this is what happens when there's a block somewhere. In this example, there's a bundle branch block, which describes when the signal can't go down one or both of the bundle branches; this usually results in these wide QRS complexes **(Figure 3.9)**.

Next, check for changes in the sequence of the waves; changes most often involve the two depolarization waves, the P wave and the QRS complex. You can make sure that there is a P wave before every QRS complex, and a QRS complex after every P wave. For example, if there's a premature ventricular contraction like this, then there may be a QRS complex *without* a preceding P wave. On the flip side, if there's a third degree AV block, then there may be a P wave that isn't followed by a QRS complex **(Figure 3.10)**.

SUMMARY

All right, let's quickly recap. One quick way to estimate the heart rate on an ECG is to remember that the heart rate is 300, 150, 100, 75, 60, or 50, depending on whether there's one, two, three, four, five, or six boxes between QRS complexes. To help identify an irregular rhythm, you can look at the morphology of the waveform, and make sure that there is a P wave before every QRS complex, and a QRS complex after every P wave **(Figure 3.11)**.

Figure 3.11

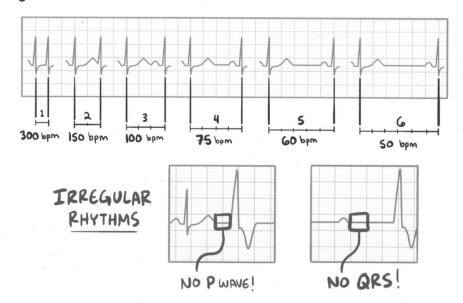

Axis

osmosis.org/learn/ecg_axis

To read an ECG, there are a few key elements to keep in mind; one is to figure out the axis **(Figure 4.1)**. The axis of an ECG is the average direction of electrical movement through the heart during a depolarization. Specifically, axis usually refers to the mean QRS vector, which is the size and direction of the depolarization wave as it moves through the ventricles. Normally, the QRS axis aims downward and to the left in relation to the body.

DEPOLARIZATION

So, if we simplify this heart a bit, normally, the sinoatrial node (SA node) sends an electrical signal that propagates outward through the walls of the heart and contracts both upper chambers **(Figure 4.2)**. Then, that signal moves to the atrioventricular (AV node) where the signal is delayed for a split second, and then goes down into the ventricles, or lower chambers. Here, it moves down the bundle of His into the left and right bundle branches, and into each ventricle's Purkinje fibers, which causes them to contract as well **(Figure 4.3)**.

Figure 4.1

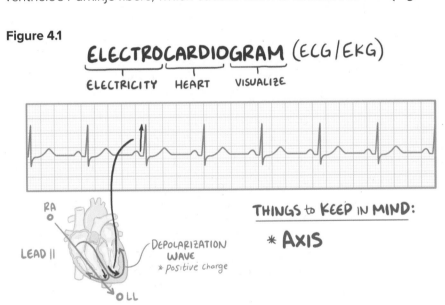

ELECTROCARDIOGRAM (ECG/EKG)

ELECTRICITY   HEART   VISUALIZE

RA

LEAD II

DEPOLARIZATION WAVE
* positive charge

LL

THINGS to KEEP IN MIND:

* AXIS

Figure 4.2

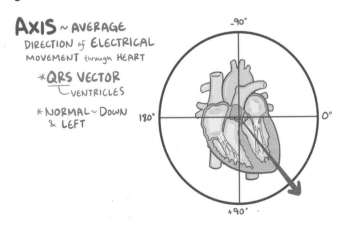

AXIS ~ AVERAGE DIRECTION of ELECTRICAL MOVEMENT through HEART

*QRS VECTOR
  VENTRICLES

* NORMAL ~ DOWN & LEFT

-90°

180°   0°

+90°

Figure 4.3

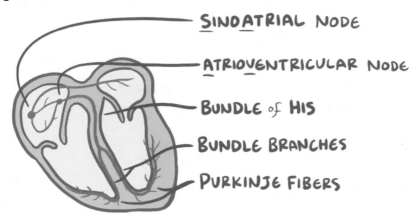

SINOATRIAL NODE

ATRIOVENTRICULAR NODE

BUNDLE of HIS

BUNDLE BRANCHES

PURKINJE FIBERS

Figure 4.4

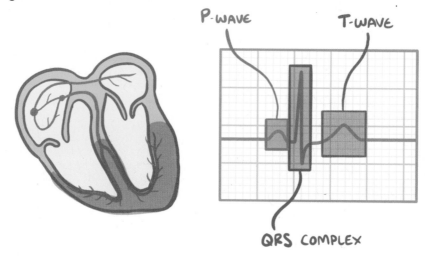

P-WAVE

T-WAVE

QRS COMPLEX

Figure 4.5

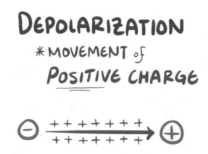

DEPOLARIZATION
* MOVEMENT of
POSITIVE CHARGE

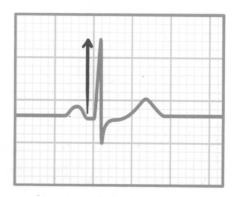

On an ECG, the atrial depolarization is seen as a P wave, the ventricular contraction is seen as a QRS complex, and the ventricular repolarization, a period of relaxation, is seen as a T wave **(Figure 4.4)**. Keep in mind that a depolarization is caused by the movement of positive charge, so if this movement of positive charge is going *toward* the positive electrode, then it's captured as a *positive* deflection on an ECG **(Figure 4.5)**.

Figure 4.6

AVERAGE QRS VECTOR

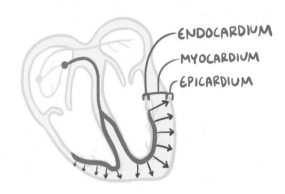

- ENDOCARDIUM
- MYOCARDIUM
- EPICARDIUM

Figure 4.7

AVERAGE QRS VECTOR

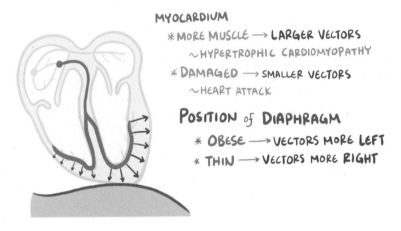

MYOCARDIUM
* MORE MUSCLE → LARGER VECTORS
  ~ HYPERTROPHIC CARDIOMYOPATHY
* DAMAGED → SMALLER VECTORS
  ~ HEART ATTACK

POSITION of DIAPHRAGM
* OBESE → VECTORS MORE LEFT
* THIN → VECTORS MORE RIGHT

MEAN QRS VECTOR

With this in mind, let's take a closer look at the mean, or average, QRS vector. After the depolarization wave arrives at the AV node, it travels down the interventricular septum and begins depolarizing the ventricles. The Purkinje fibers sit just below the endocardium, the innermost layer of the heart. After the endocardium, there's the myocardium, the cardiac muscle cells, and finally, the epicardium, which is the outer layer. Therefore, each Purkinje fiber initiates a depolarization vector that travels directly outward; it starts in the endocardium, goes through the myocardium, and ends in the epicardium **(Figure 4.6)**. Because they transmit a depolarization wave so quickly, they all fire off pretty much in unison. The more muscle tissue in the myocardial layer that a vector has to travel through, the large the size of the vector. So, as with hypertrophic cardiomyopathy, where the heart muscle gets thicker, you get bigger vectors.

However, if the heart tissue has been damaged, such as from a heart attack, then you have smaller vectors because the heart cells can't depolarize anymore. The position of the diaphragm can also affect vectors because it's usually sort of sitting right up against the heart. In obese people the diaphragm gets pushed upwards, rotating the heart further to the left. In thin people, the diaphragm lowers, rotating the heart a bit the other way **(Figure 4.7)**.

Figure 4.8

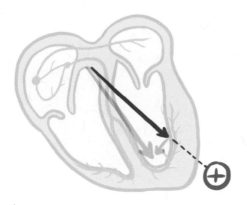
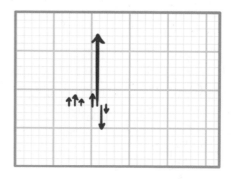

Figure 4.9

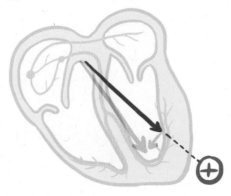
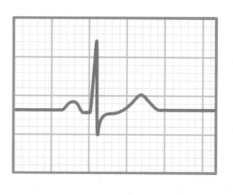

Figure 4.10

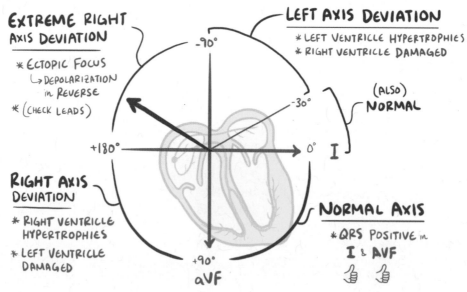

Figure 4.11

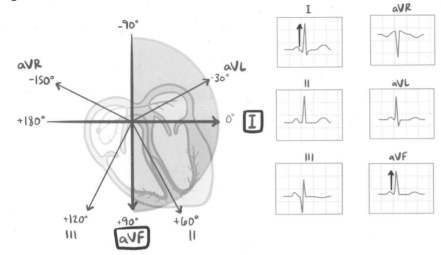

Figure 4.12

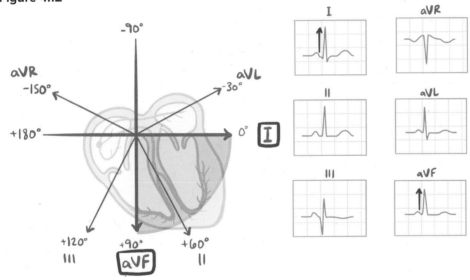

Figure 4.13

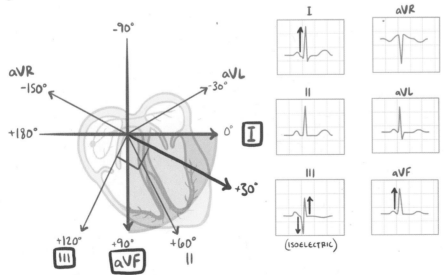

Figure 4.14

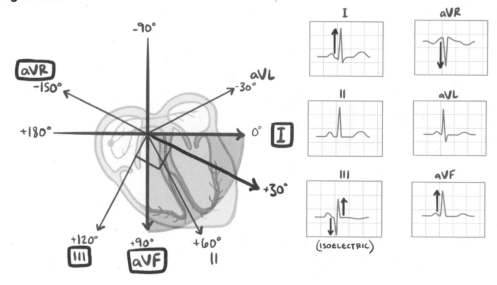

Figure 4.15

CHEST LEADS

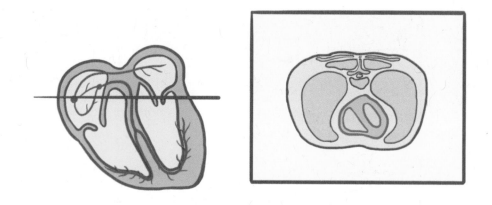

Figure 4.16

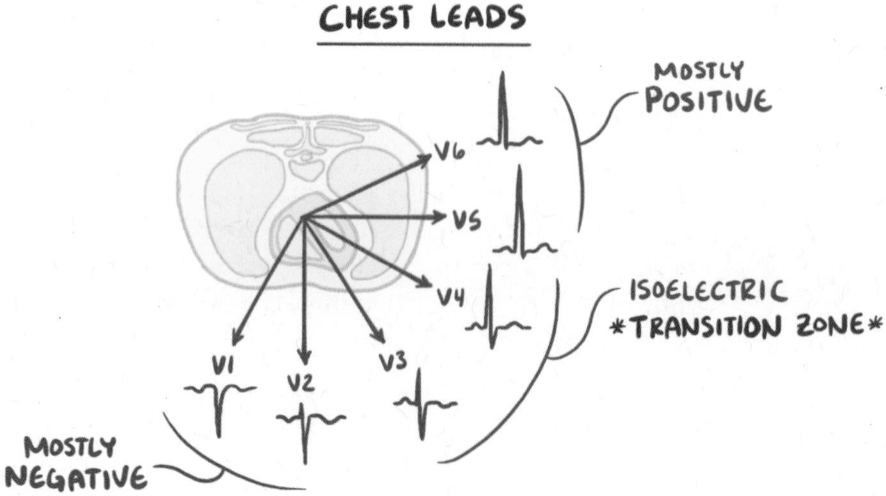

CHEST LEADS

Figure 4.17

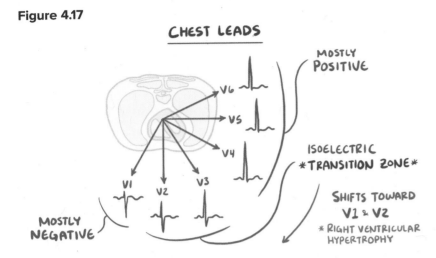

When everything is taken into consideration and all of the individual vectors are added up, there's one overall representative vector arrow, which starts from the AV node and points in one direction through the ventricles **(Figure 4.8)**. Now, vectors can be broken down into two perpendicular vector components, so if you look at the component pointing at the positive lead electrode, that's what is recorded on the ECG. Therefore, when you plot these vectors over the course of ventricular depolarization, the QRS complex emerges **(Figure 4.9)**.

All right, to figure out the direction of the axis we can start by looking at lead I and aVF. Lead I moves from right to left across the heart, so anything pointing to the left will be positive in lead I; in contrast, aVF points downward, so any vector pointing downward will be positive in aVF. So, looking at our overall vector from before, it's pointing both down and to the left, and both are positive. Thus, it's in the bottom left quadrant between 0 and +90 degrees; that's a normal axis. If it's up in lead I and aVF, you can imagine it's like seeing two thumbs up, which means that everything is okay! If the vector is positive in lead I and negative in aVF, then it's in this quadrant; it could be normal if it's between 0 and -30 degrees. However, if it's between -30 and -90, it could be considered left axis deviation. Left axis deviation can happen when the left ventricle hypertrophies, or when the right ventricle becomes damaged and loses healthy tissue. If the opposite happens, and the vector is negative in lead I and positive in aVF, then it's in this quadrant between +90 and +180 degrees; we call this right axis deviation. Right axis deviation can happen when the right ventricle hypertrophies, or when the left ventricle is damaged and loses healthy tissue. Finally, if the vector is negative in both lead I and aVF, then it's a very rare case called extreme right axis deviation between -90 and +180 degrees. This can sometimes happen when there's an ectopic focus that causes depolarization to start from the bottom of the ventricles, and travel in the reverse direction. It's also a good idea to double check that the leads are placed correctly **(Figure 4.10)**.

You can figure out the QRS vector within 30 degrees by looking at someone's ECGs. Specifically, to do so, you'll look at the six leads, I, II, III, aVR, aVL, and aVF, which correspond to 0 degrees, +60 degrees, +120 degrees, -150, -30, and +90, respectively **(Figure 4.11)**. Here, lead I is clearly positive, which means that the axis is somewhere over here, and lead aVF is positive; this puts the axis in the lower left quadrant between 0 and +90 degrees, which is a normal axis **(Figure 4.12)**. To be more precise, it looks like lead III is the closest to being isoelectric, which means equal positive and negative deflections; therefore, lead III must actually run *perpendicular* to the QRS vector, so 120 degrees subtract 90 degrees is the +30 degree line **(Figure 4.13)**. Notice that this happens to sit on the same line as aVR, but in the opposite direction **(Figure 4.14)**. We would think that this vector should look *negative* in aVR, and it does!

Figure 4.18

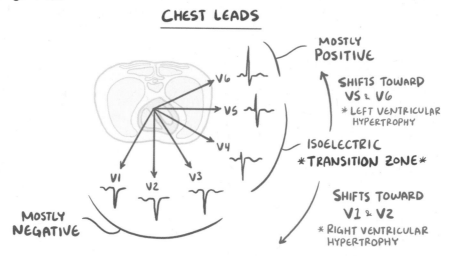

CHEST LEADS

MOSTLY POSITIVE

SHIFTS TOWARD V5 & V6
* LEFT VENTRICULAR HYPERTROPHY

ISOELECTRIC
TRANSITION ZONE

SHIFTS TOWARD V1 & V2
* RIGHT VENTRICULAR HYPERTROPHY

MOSTLY NEGATIVE

Now, let's switch gears and talk about the chest leads, which essentially view the heart in a different plane **(Figure 4.15)**. Looking down at the heart we have leads V_1, V_2, V_3, V_4, V_5, and V_6. Normally, the QRS complex is negative in leads V_1 and V_2, isoelectric in lead V_3 and V_4, which is called the transition zone, and positive in leads V_5 and V_6 **(Figure 4.16)**. If the transition zone shifts toward V_1 or V_2, and looks isoelectric instead of negative, it suggests that the heart may be rotated to the person's right, which can happen if the right ventricle is hypertrophied **(Figure 4.17)**. On the other hand, if leads V_5 or V_6 look isoelectric instead of positive, it suggests that the heart may be rotated to the person's left, which can happen if the left ventricle is hypertrophied **(Figure 4.18)**.

SUMMARY

All right, let's quickly recap. A normal heart's axis is between -30 and +90 degrees. Right ventricular hypertrophy can cause the axis to be between +90 and +180, and can sometimes cause the V_1 and V_2 chest leads to appear isoelectric. Left ventricular hypertrophy can cause the axis to be between -30 and -90, and can sometimes cause the V_5 and V_6 chest leads to appear isoelectric **(Figure 4.19)**.

Figure 4.19

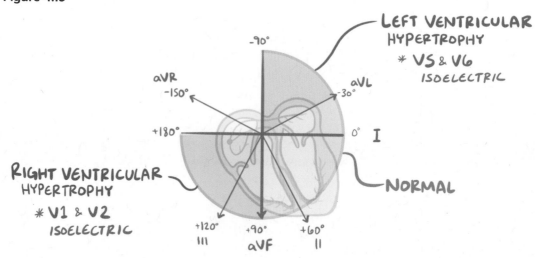

LEFT VENTRICULAR HYPERTROPHY
* V5 & V6 ISOELECTRIC

-90°

aVR -150°

aVL -30°

+180°

0° I

NORMAL

RIGHT VENTRICULAR HYPERTROPHY
* V1 & V2 ISOELECTRIC

+120° III

+90° aVF

+60° II

Intervals

osmosis.org/learn/ecg_intervals

When reading an ECG, there are a few key elements to keep in mind; one of them is looking at the intervals **(Figure 5.1)**. In a typical waveform, there's a P wave, QRS complex, and T wave. In addition, there are certain intervals, including the PR interval, the QRS complex itself, and the QT interval.

Figure 5.1

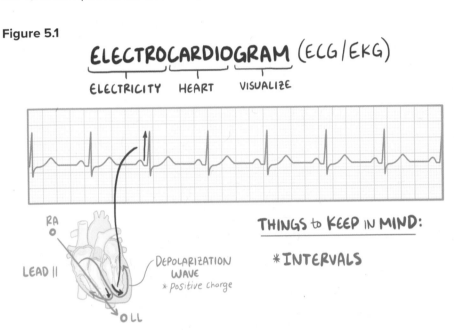

ELECTROCARDIOGRAM (ECG/EKG)

ELECTRICITY   HEART   VISUALIZE

RA

LEAD II

DEPOLARIZATION WAVE
* positive charge

O LL

THINGS to KEEP IN MIND:

* INTERVALS

Figure 5.2

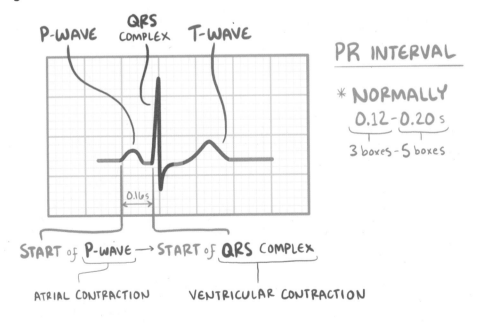

P-WAVE   QRS COMPLEX   T-WAVE

0.16s

START of P-WAVE → START of QRS COMPLEX

ATRIAL CONTRACTION   VENTRICULAR CONTRACTION

PR INTERVAL

* NORMALLY
  0.12 - 0.20 s
  3 boxes - 5 boxes

Figure 5.3

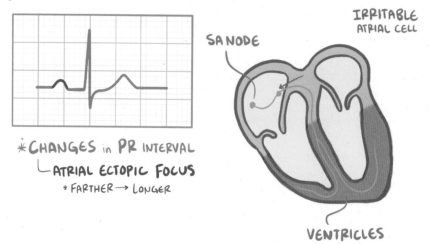

* CHANGES in PR INTERVAL
  └ ATRIAL ECTOPIC FOCUS
    * FARTHER → LONGER

Figure 5.4

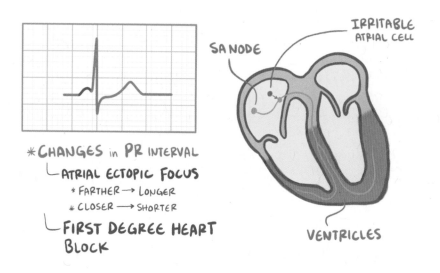

* CHANGES in PR INTERVAL
  └ ATRIAL ECTOPIC FOCUS
    * FARTHER → LONGER
    * CLOSER → SHORTER
  └ FIRST DEGREE HEART BLOCK

Figure 5.5

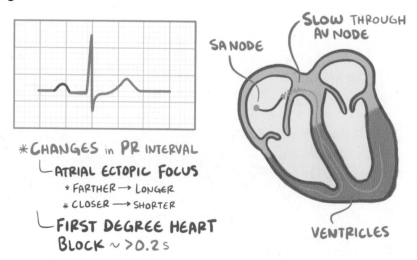

* CHANGES in PR INTERVAL
  └ ATRIAL ECTOPIC FOCUS
    * FARTHER → LONGER
    * CLOSER → SHORTER
  └ FIRST DEGREE HEART BLOCK ~ >0.2 s

Figure 5.6

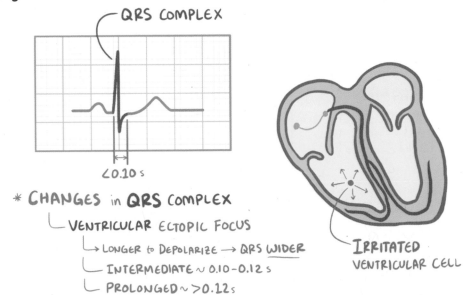

QRS COMPLEX

<0.10 s

* CHANGES in **QRS** COMPLEX

└ VENTRICULAR ECTOPIC FOCUS

└→ LONGER to DEPOLARIZE → QRS WIDER

└ INTERMEDIATE ~ 0.10-0.12 s

└ PROLONGED ~ >0.12 s

IRRITATED
VENTRICULAR CELL

PR INTERVAL

The PR interval spans from the beginning of the P wave to the beginning of the QRS complex, and it represents the time from the beginning of atrial depolarization to the beginning of ventricular depolarization. It's normally 0.12-0.20 seconds, which is three to five little boxes, since each little box is 0.04 seconds. Therefore, the PR interval shown is about four boxes or 0.16 seconds **(Figure 5.2)**.

Any deviation in the normal depolarization pathway from the SA node to the ventricles can change the PR interval. For example, consider if the atria are depolarized by an ectopic atrial focus, such as an irritable atrial cell outside of the SA node. If it was farther away from the AV node, it'd result in a *longer* PR interval, because the signal has to travel a greater distance **(Figure 5.3)**.

Alternatively, if it was really *close* to the AV node, the PR interval might be super short. Another example is first degree heart block, which is when the electrical signal travels more slowly through the AV node than it normally does, causing the PR interval to lengthen beyond 0.2 seconds **(Figure 5.4)**.

QRS COMPLEX

The QRS complex represents depolarization of the ventricles; it's normally less than 100 milliseconds or two and a half little boxes. Just like the PR interval, the QRS duration can differ in its path from the AV node to the ventricles **(Figure 5.5)**.

For example, if an ectopic ventricular focus, such as an irritated ventricular cell, fires off, the resulting depolarization wave will move slowly from muscle cell to muscle cell, instead of traveling quickly through the electrical conduction system. Therefore, it takes a longer time to depolarize the ventricles, and the QRS is wider. It's considered intermediate if it's 100 to 120 milliseconds, and prolonged if it's over 120 milliseconds, or three little boxes **(Figure 5.6)**.

Figure 5.7

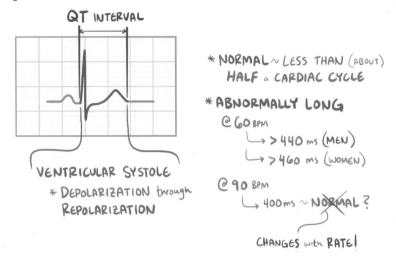

QT INTERVAL

* NORMAL ~ LESS THAN (ABOUT) HALF a CARDIAC CYCLE

* ABNORMALLY LONG

@ 60 BPM
→ > 440 ms (MEN)
→ > 460 ms (WOMEN)

@ 90 BPM
→ 400 ms ~ NORMAL?

CHANGES with RATE!

VENTRICULAR SYSTOLE
* DEPOLARIZATION through REPOLARIZATION

Figure 5.8

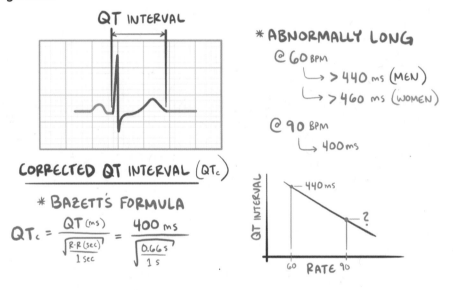

QT INTERVAL

CORRECTED QT INTERVAL (QTc)

* BAZETT'S FORMULA

$$QT_c = \frac{QT\,(ms)}{\sqrt{\frac{R\text{-}R\,(sec)}{1\,sec}}} = \frac{400\,ms}{\sqrt{\frac{0.66\,s}{1\,s}}}$$

* ABNORMALLY LONG

@ 60 BPM
→ > 440 ms (MEN)
→ > 460 ms (WOMEN)

@ 90 BPM
→ 400 ms

440 ms

?

QT INTERVAL / 60 RATE 90

Figure 5.9

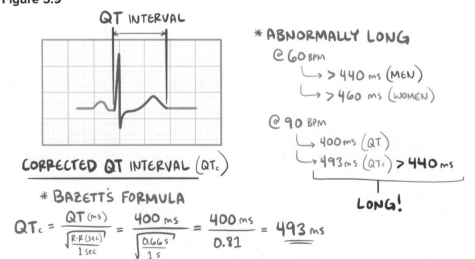

QT INTERVAL

CORRECTED QT INTERVAL (QTc)

* BAZETT'S FORMULA

$$QT_c = \frac{QT\,(ms)}{\sqrt{\frac{R\text{-}R\,(sec)}{1\,sec}}} = \frac{400\,ms}{\sqrt{\frac{0.66\,s}{1\,s}}} = \frac{400\,ms}{0.81} = \underline{493\,ms}$$

* ABNORMALLY LONG

@ 60 BPM
→ > 440 ms (MEN)
→ > 460 ms (WOMEN)

@ 90 BPM
→ 400 ms (QT)
→ 493 ms (QTc) > 440 ms

LONG!

Figure 5.10

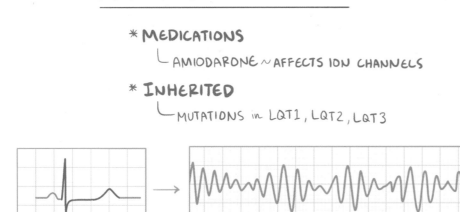

PROLONGED QT INTERVAL

* MEDICATIONS
  └ AMIODARONE ~ AFFECTS ION CHANNELS

* INHERITED
  └ MUTATIONS in LQT1, LQT2, LQT3

LONG QT   →   TORSADES DE POINTES

QT INTERVAL

The QT interval spans from the beginning of the QRS complex to the end of the T wave. It represents ventricular systole, which is the entire span from depolarization through repolarization. Normally, the QT interval should be less than half of a cardiac cycle. In fact, for a heart rate of 60 beats per minute, the QT interval is generally considered to be abnormally long when it's greater than 440 milliseconds in men, or 460 milliseconds in women. If you measure someone's QT interval at a different rate, say 90 beats per minute, and it was 400 milliseconds, you might think that that'd be considered normal; however, you can't really use these values to compare to the normal QT interval at 60 beats per minute, or bpm, because the QT interval changes depending on the rate **(Figure 5.7)**.

As rate increases, the QT interval decreases; thus, at 60 bpm, the abnormal cutoff might be 440 ms, whereas at 90 bpm, it's likely something lower. So, what we have to do is find the *corrected* QT interval, or QT$_c$, at the different rate. Then, you can compare it to the QT interval at 60 beats per minute. Even though there are several formulas you can use, Bazett's formula is probably the simplest, where the corrected QT interval equals the QT interval in milliseconds, divided by the square root of the R to R interval in seconds, divided by one second. As a side-note, this formula is usually expressed *without* the "divide by 1 second" part, but the astute observer will notice that the units won't work out if you leave it out **(Figure 5.8)**.

Let's use our 90 bpm and 400 milliseconds QT interval from before, and imagine the person is male. If we plug in 400 for QT and 90 beats per minute, or .66 seconds per beat, we have a QT of 400 milliseconds divided by the square root of 0.66 seconds over 1 second, which is 400 milliseconds divided by 0.81, which is unitless, and we get a corrected QT interval of 493 milliseconds. Now we can compare this sum to the value at 60 bpm. We see that the corrected QTc is actually *greater* than 440 ms, which means that this measured QT interval of 400 ms at 90 bpm is indeed abnormally long **(Figure 5.9)**!

The QT interval can be prolonged by medications, such as amiodarone, which is an antiarrhythmic that affects cardiomyocyte ion channels, or caused by inherited long QT syndromes, where there are mutations in genes, including LQT1, LQT2, or LQT3. One of the most feared complications of having a prolonged QT interval is a type of ventricular tachycardia called torsades de pointes, which can lead to sudden cardiac death; here, the ECG shows a "twisting of the points" **(Figure 5.10)**.

Figure 5.11

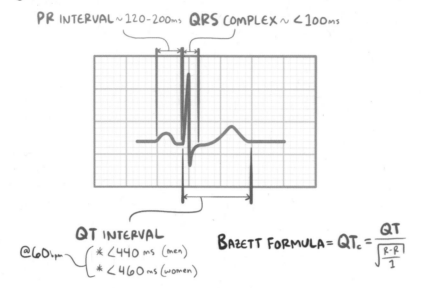

PR INTERVAL ~ 120-200ms   QRS COMPLEX ~ < 100ms

QT INTERVAL

@60bpm { * < 440 ms (men)
        { * < 460 ms (women)

BAZETT FORMULA = $QT_c = \dfrac{QT}{\sqrt{\dfrac{R-R}{1}}}$

SUMMARY

All right, let's quickly recap. An ECG waveform has a PR interval that's usually 120 to 200 milliseconds, a QRS complex that's less than 100 milliseconds, and a QT interval that's less than 440 milliseconds in men and 460 milliseconds in women; these values are for rates at 60 bpm. Bazett's formula can be used to find the corrected QT interval, which you can use to compare rates other than 60 bpm to the normal rate **(Figure 5.11)**.

QRS Transition

osmosis.org/learn/ecg_qrs_transition

To read an ECG, there are a few key elements to keep in mind; one is to figure out the QRS transition (**Figure 6.1**).The chest leads (**Figure 6.2**) will have a mostly positive deflection, if a depolarization wave is moving towards them.

QRS VECTOR & TRANSITION ZONE

The QRS transition zone refers to where the QRS complex switches from being mostly negative to mostly positive, from the point of view of the chest leads, V_1 through V_6, which "view" the heart through the horizontal plane. The QRS transition usually happens in lead V_3 or V_4, depending on factors such as chest lead placement and the exact anatomy of a person's heart (**Figure 6.3**). So, the QRS transition tells us when the overall QRS vector is aligned in the direction of the chest leads; it's a way of understanding what's happening to the QRS axis in the horizontal plane.

Figure 6.1

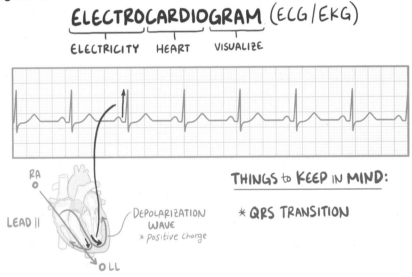

Figure 6.2

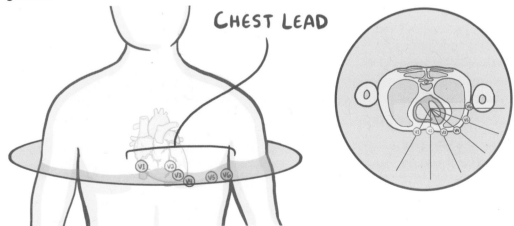

Figure 6.3

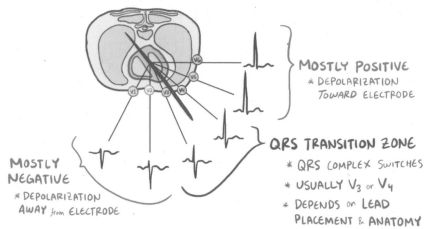

CHEST LEADS

MOSTLY POSITIVE
* DEPOLARIZATION
  TOWARD ELECTRODE

MOSTLY NEGATIVE
* DEPOLARIZATION
  AWAY from ELECTRODE

QRS TRANSITION ZONE
* QRS COMPLEX SWITCHES
* USUALLY V$_3$ or V$_4$
* DEPENDS on LEAD
  PLACEMENT & ANATOMY

Figure 6.4

QRS TRANSITION ZONE **SHIFTS**

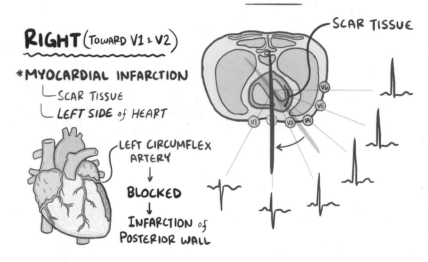

RIGHT (TOWARD V1 & V2)

* MYOCARDIAL INFARCTION
  └ SCAR TISSUE
  └ LEFT SIDE of HEART

LEFT CIRCUMFLEX ARTERY
↓
BLOCKED
↓
INFARCTION of POSTERIOR WALL

SCAR TISSUE

Figure 6.5

QRS TRANSITION ZONE **SHIFTS**

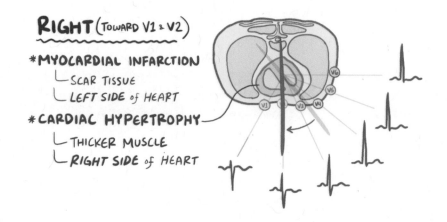

RIGHT (TOWARD V1 & V2)

* MYOCARDIAL INFARCTION
  └ SCAR TISSUE
  └ LEFT SIDE of HEART
* CARDIAC HYPERTROPHY
  └ THICKER MUSCLE
  └ RIGHT SIDE of HEART

Figure 6.6

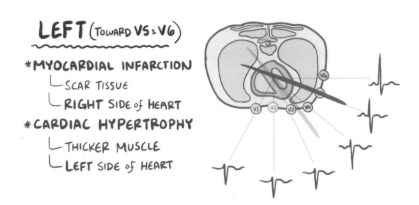

If something alters the heart's overall QRS vector, then the QRS transition zone can shift to the right, towards V_1 and V_2, or to the left, towards V_5 and V_6. For example, a myocardial infarction leads to the formation of scar tissue that can't depolarize. Generally speaking, the QRS transition zone will shift away from a region of scar tissue, because it no longer contributes to the overall QRS vector. Consider the following: a blockage in the left circumflex artery can cause infarction of the posterior wall of the left ventricle, which would lead to a rightward rotation of the QRS transition zone, toward V_1 and V_2 **(Figure 6.4)**. Another example would be cardiac hypertrophy, because a thicker muscular wall contributes more to the overall QRS vector **(Figure 6.5)**. If it's right ventricular hypertrophy, it would lead to a rightward rotation of the QRS transition zone, towards V_1 and V_2, similar to the result of an infarction of the posterior wall of the left ventricle. In contrast, a right ventricular infarction or a left ventricular hypertrophy would lead to a leftward rotation of the QRS transition zone, towards V_5 and V_6 **(Figure 6.6)**.

SUMMARY

All right, let's quickly recap. The QRS transition zone, in the horizontal plane, is where the QRS complex switches from being mostly negative to mostly positive; it normally happens in lead V_3 or V_4. The QRS transition zone rotates away from previous myocardial infarctions, and toward hypertrophied tissue **(Figure 6.7)**.

Figure 6.7

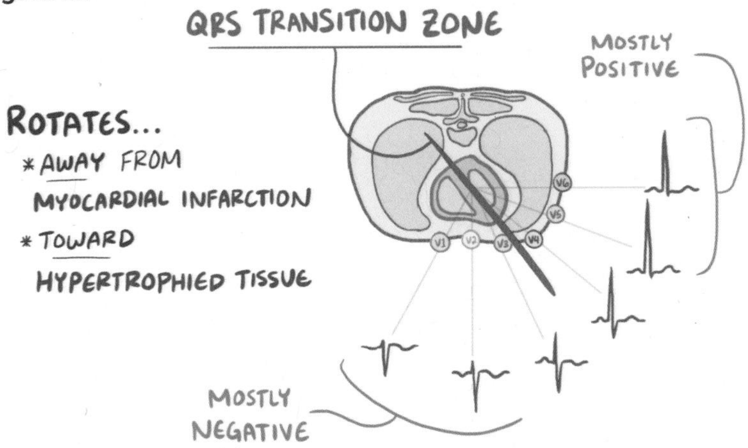

Cardiac Hypertrophy & Enlargement

osmosis.org/learn/ecg_cardiac_hypertrophy_and_enlargement

There are lots of things to look for when reading an ECG, including figuring out if part of the heart has undergone hypertrophy or enlargement **(Figure 7.1)**. *Hypertrophy* means that a heart's muscular wall has increased in thickness. *Dilation* refers to an increase in the volume of the chamber. The term *enlargement* is generally used when both hypertrophy and dilation occur together; this is what typically happens in the atria. In contrast, the ventricles often undergo hypertrophy without dilation **(Figure 7.2)**. An ECG can show evidence of hypertrophy and enlargement in all of the heart's four chambers. Let's go through them one by one.

ATRIAL ENLARGEMENT

Normally, atrial depolarization produces a pretty normal-looking symmetric P wave. In right atrial enlargement, all of that extra right atrial muscle tissue results in a large P wave in leads V_1 and V_2 that is often over 1.5 mm, as well as in the inferior leads, which are leads II, III, and aVF, that is often over 2.5 mm. One reason why right atrial enlargement develops is that there can be a stenotic, or narrowed, tricuspid valve that makes it more difficult for the atria to eject blood into the ventricles. In response, the right atrium enlarges **(Figure 7.3; Figure 7.4)**.

In left atrial enlargement, the left atrium has extra muscle tissue that results in a P wave with two peaks in lead II. The entire wave stretches out over 110 ms, and has a gap of over 40 ms separating the two peaks. In lead V_1, the P wave is biphasic, which means that it looks like a hill with a valley alongside it. The negative portion is usually 1 mm deep, and lasts for more than 40 ms. Left atrial enlargement also develops from a stenotic valve, but this time it's the mitral valve that causes the left atrium to get bigger **(Figure 7.5)**.

Figure 7.1

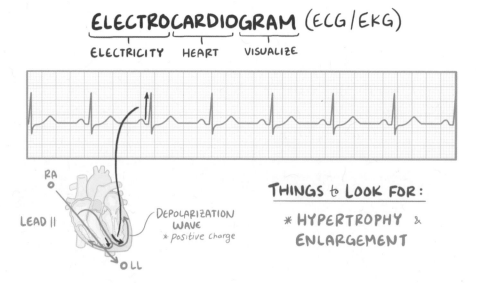

ELECTROCARDIOGRAM (ECG/EKG)

ELECTRICITY   HEART   VISUALIZE

RA
LEAD II
DEPOLARIZATION WAVE
* Positive charge
LL

THINGS to LOOK FOR:
* HYPERTROPHY & ENLARGEMENT

Figure 7.2

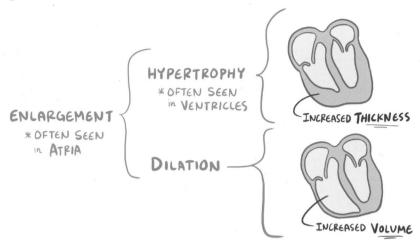

Figure 7.3

RIGHT ATRIAL ENLARGEMENT

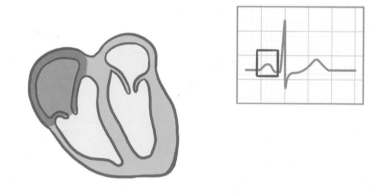

Figure 7.4

LEFT ATRIAL ENLARGEMENT

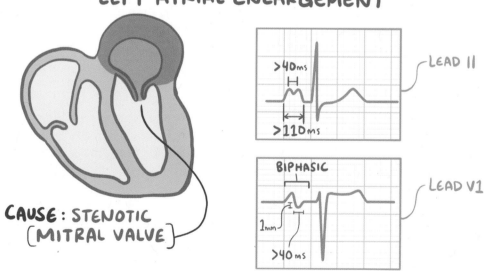

Figure 7.5

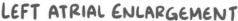

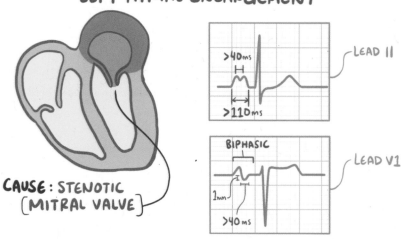

LEFT ATRIAL ENLARGEMENT

LEAD II

>40ms

>110ms

BIPHASIC

LEAD V1

1mm

>40 ms

CAUSE: STENOTIC (MITRAL VALVE)

Figure 7.6

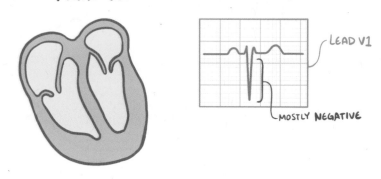

RIGHT VENTRICULAR HYPERTROPHY

LEAD V1

MOSTLY NEGATIVE

VENTRICULAR HYPERTROPHY

Normally, the QRS complex is mostly negative in lead V_1, because the large left ventricle, which carries the greatest amount of muscle tissue, is oriented down and away from this electrode **(Figure 7.6)**.

In right ventricular hypertrophy, the thicker right ventricle helps to counterbalance the left ventricle and makes lead V_1 more positive. Specifically, it makes the R wave bigger, which is the upward deflection of the QRS complex. In fact, a dominant R wave in V_1 is a classic sign of right ventricular hypertrophy; it's defined as an R wave that is over 7 mm tall, or 7 little boxes, and is larger than the S wave, making the R/S ratio > 1. Another classic sign of right ventricular hypertrophy is a dominant S wave in V_5 or V_6, meaning that it's over 7 mm deep, or 7 little boxes, and bigger than the R wave, making the R/S ratio < 1. Typically, there's also right axis deviation in right ventricular hypertrophy that results in an axis of 110 degrees or more **(Figure 7.7)**. In right ventricular hypertrophy the QRS complex is <120 ms, meaning that it's not longer than normal. This is important because it means that the changes can't be the result of something like a right bundle branch block, which would cause a prolonged QRS complex. Right ventricular hypertrophy can develop for a number of reasons. A common cause is pulmonary hypertension, which makes sense because the right ventricle has to build up muscle to push blood into the lungs **(Figure 7.8)**.

Figure 7.7

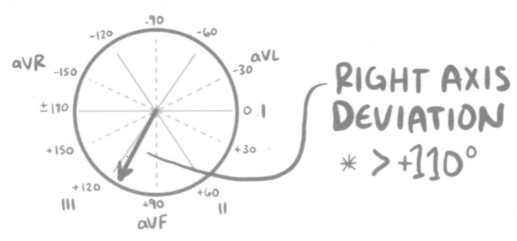

RIGHT AXIS DEVIATION
* > +110°

Figure 7.8

RIGHT VENTRICULAR HYPERTROPHY

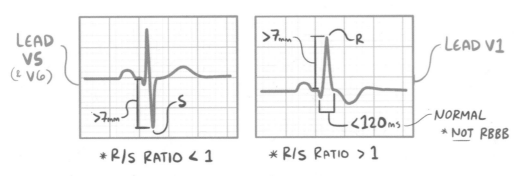

LEAD V5 (& V6)

>7mm
S

* R/S RATIO < 1

>7mm
R
LEAD V1
<120ms
NORMAL
* NOT RBBB

* R/S RATIO > 1

CAUSE: PULMONARY HYPERTENSION

Figure 7.9

LEFT VENTRICULAR HYPERTROPHY

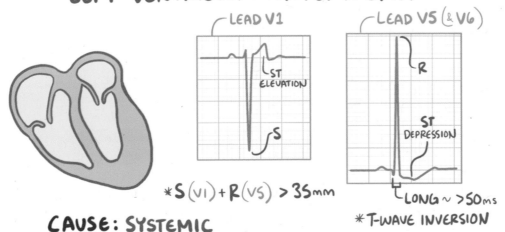

LEAD V1
ST ELEVATION
S

LEAD V5 (& V6)
R
ST DEPRESSION
LONG ~ >50ms
* T-WAVE INVERSION

* S(V1) + R(V5) > 35mm

CAUSE: SYSTEMIC HYPERTENSION

In left ventricular hypertrophy, the pattern is almost the opposite of what happens in right ventricular hypertrophy. Lead V_1 has even more positive charge traveling away from it than usual, making the S wave really deep. Meanwhile, lead V_5 and V_6 are located on the side of the left ventricle, and therefore have an enormous R wave. The most commonly used voltage criteria to identify left ventricular hypertrophy is that the sum of the S wave in V_1 and the tallest R wave in V_5 or V_6 has to be over 35 millimeters, or 35 little boxes. Additional criteria include having an R wave that goes on for longer than usual, typically over 50 ms, and ST elevation in V_1, ST segment depression, and T wave inversion in V_5 or V_6. These are signs that the left ventricle is straining during muscle contraction. Left ventricular hypertrophy commonly develops due to systemic hypertension, or elevated systemic blood pressure, because the left ventricle needs more muscle so that it can eject blood against higher pressures **(Figure 7.9)**.

SUMMARY

All right, let's quickly recap. Right atrial enlargement shows a big P wave in lead II and V_1, whereas left atrial enlargement has a biphasic P wave in lead V_1 and a double-humped P wave in lead II. Right ventricular hypertrophy shows a big R wave in V_1 and a big S wave in V_5 and V_6, whereas left ventricular hypertrophy shows the opposite: an enormous S wave in V_1 and a large R wave in V_5 and V_6 that add up to over 35 mm **(Figure 7.10)**.

Figure 7.10

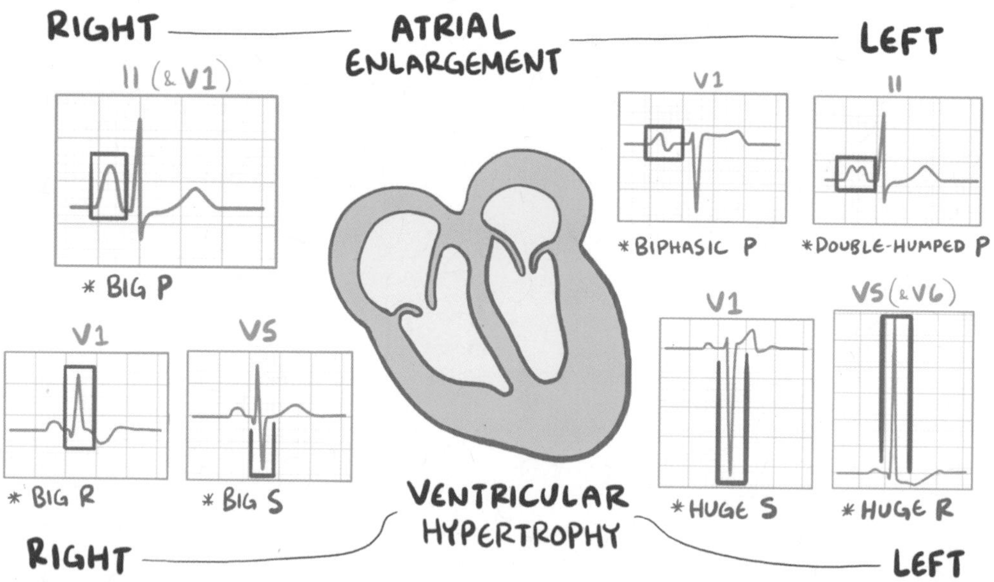

Cardiac Infarction & Ischemia

osmosis.org/learn/ecg_cardiac_infarction_and_ischemia

To read an ECG, there are a few key elements to keep in mind; one is to figure out if part of the heart is suffering from ischemia or has undergone an infarction **(Figure 8.1)**. The term *ischemia* means that blood flow to tissue has decreased, which results in *hypoxia*, or insufficient oxygen in the tissue. *Infarction* goes one step further, because it means that blood flow has been completely cut off, which results in necrosis, or cellular death. This typically happens if blood flow has been cut off for about 20 minutes **(Figure 8.2)**.

In the heart, ischemia and infarction can be transmural, affecting the entire thickness of the myocardium, or subendocardial, affecting just the innermost part of the myocardium, the part just beneath the endocardium. Out of the four chambers of the heart, the ECG is most sensitive to transmural and subendocardial ischemia or infarction in the left ventricle because that's the chamber with the thickest walls; in other words, it has the most cardiac tissue **(Figure 8.3)**.

Figure 8.1

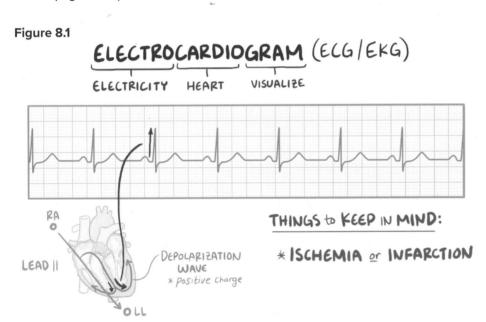

Figure 8.2

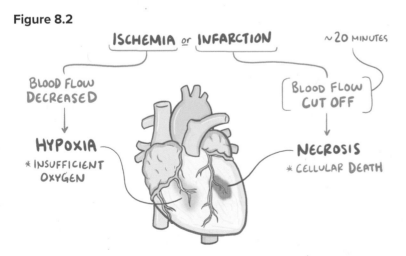

Figure 8.3

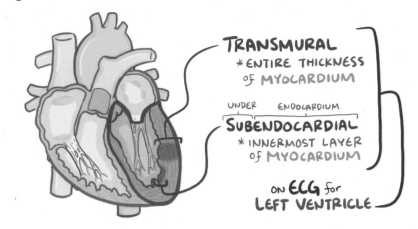

TRANSMURAL
* ENTIRE THICKNESS
  of MYOCARDIUM

UNDER   ENDOCARDIUM
SUBENDOCARDIAL
* INNERMOST LAYER
  of MYOCARDIUM

ON ECG for
LEFT VENTRICLE

Figure 8.4

SUBENDOCARDIAL ISCHEMIA

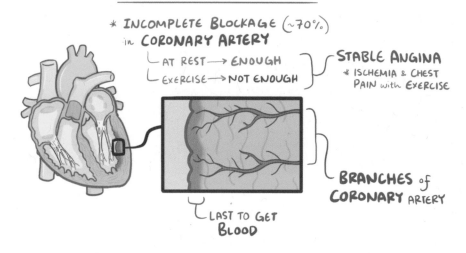

* INCOMPLETE BLOCKAGE (~70%)
  in CORONARY ARTERY
  └ AT REST → ENOUGH
  └ EXERCISE → NOT ENOUGH

STABLE ANGINA
* ISCHEMIA & CHEST
  PAIN with EXERCISE

BRANCHES of
CORONARY ARTERY

LAST TO GET
BLOOD

Figure 8.5

SUBENDOCARDIAL ISCHEMIA

* ST DEPRESSION *
  └ J-POINT DOWN by ≥ 0.5mm

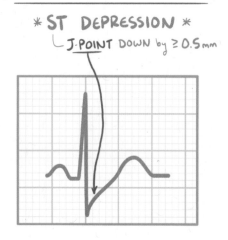

Figure 8.6

SUBENDOCARDIAL ISCHEMIA

* ST DEPRESSION *
└ J·POINT DOWN by ≥ 0.5mm

UPWARD-SLOPING   DOWNWARD-SLOPING   HORIZONTAL

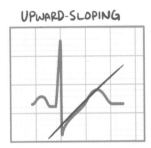 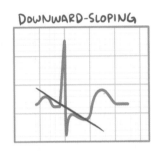 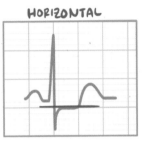

* OFTEN AFFECTS **LEADS** I, II, V4, V5, V6
└ DIFFICULT to DETERMINE **ARTERY** INVOLVED

SUBENDOCARDIAL ISCHEMIA

Subendocardial ischemia might happen when there's incomplete blockage, let's say 70%, in a coronary artery. In this situation, there's enough blood flowing through to meet the demand of the myocardium when the person is at rest, but during exercise, there's not enough to meet the increased demand of the myocardium. Therefore, the subendocardial tissue becomes ischemic because it's the last bit of tissue to receive blood from the tiny branches of the coronary arteries as they make their way through the ventricular wall, from outside to inside. This condition is called stable angina, because there's ischemia that causes chest pain with exercise, and the pain disappears with rest **(Figure 8.4)**.

When there's subendocardial ischemia in a region, it causes ST depressions in the corresponding lead on the ECG. An ST depression describes when the J point, which is where the QRS complex meets the ST segment, goes down by at least 0.5 mm or ½ of a small box **(Figure 8.5)**. The ST depression can be upward sloping, downward sloping, or horizontal. In subendocardial ischemia, ST depressions are usually widespread, and often affect leads I, II, and V_4 to V_6. With such widespread involvement, it's difficult to determine which coronary artery caused the ST depression **(Figure 8.6)**. As a side note, if the ST segment is depressed and curved, it may be due to the *digitalis effect*, which happens when the patient takes the medication digoxin, rather than being due to subendocardial ischemia **(Figure 8.7)**.

TRANSMURAL ISCHEMIA

Next, there's transmural ischemia. When a coronary artery is narrowed from an atherosclerotic plaque buildup over time, there are two parts to the plaque: a hard fibrous cap and the soft cheese-like interior. As blood flows past the plaque, the fibrous cap can sometimes rip. That cheesy interior is considered thrombogenic, meaning that blood clots form on it very quickly; these can quickly stop blood flow! This means that *none* of that wall gets adequate blood flow. It happens during unstable angina or during a non-ST elevation myocardial infarction, or NSTEMI for short. The key difference is that in an NSTEMI, the ischemia is so severe that damaged heart cells leak out certain enzymes, such as troponin and CK-MB **(Figure 8.8)**.

Figure 8.7

SUBENDOCARDIAL ISCHEMIA

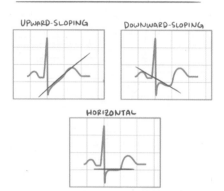

UPWARD-SLOPING   DOWNWARD-SLOPING

HORIZONTAL

DIGITALIS EFFECT

* from TAKING DIGOXIN

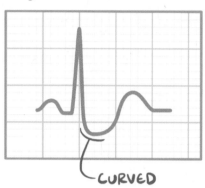

└ CURVED

Figure 8.8

TRANSMURAL ISCHEMIA

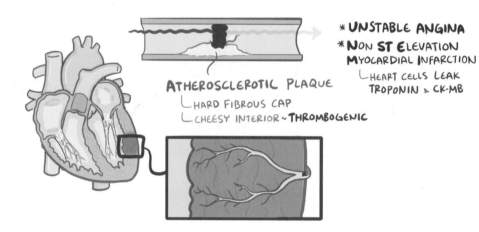

ATHEROSCLEROTIC PLAQUE
└ HARD FIBROUS CAP
└ CHEESY INTERIOR ~ **THROMBOGENIC**

* **UNSTABLE ANGINA**
* **NON ST ELEVATION**
  MYOCARDIAL INFARCTION
  └ HEART CELLS LEAK
  TROPONIN & CK-MB

Figure 8.9

TRANSMURAL ISCHEMIA

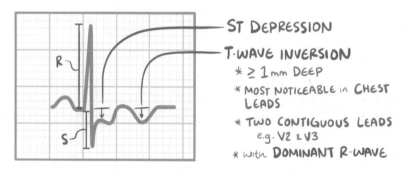

R

S

ST DEPRESSION

T-WAVE INVERSION
* ≥ 1 mm DEEP
* MOST NOTICEABLE in CHEST LEADS
* TWO CONTIGUOUS LEADS
  e.g. V2 & V3
* with DOMINANT R-WAVE

T-WAVE INVERSION
* NORMAL in III, aVR, & V1
* ABNORMAL in V2-V6

Figure 8.10

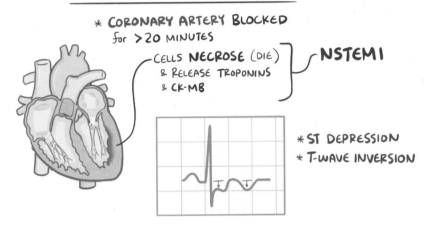

SUBENDOCARDIAL INFARCTION

* CORONARY ARTERY BLOCKED for >20 MINUTES

CELLS **NECROSE** (DIE) & RELEASE TROPONINS & CK-MB — **NSTEMI**

* ST DEPRESSION
* T-WAVE INVERSION

Figure 8.11

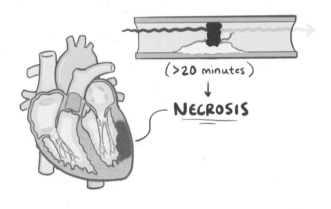

TRANSMURAL INFARCTION

(>20 minutes)

↓

NECROSIS

Figure 8.12

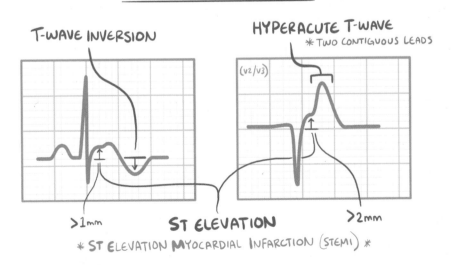

TRANSMURAL INFARCTION

T-WAVE INVERSION

HYPERACUTE T-WAVE
* TWO CONTIGUOUS LEADS

(V2/V3)

>1mm   **ST ELEVATION**   >2mm

* ST ELEVATION MYOCARDIAL INFARCTION (STEMI) *

On an ECG, both unstable angina and NSTEMI's may show ST depressions and T wave inversions. These ST depressions look similar to the ones in subendocardial ischemia. The T wave inversions are usually symmetrical, and are at least 1 mm, or 1 little box deep. They are most noticeable in the chest leads, but can also appear in the limb leads. They also have to occur in at least two contiguous leads. For example, lead V_2 and V_3 are contiguous, but leads V_3 and V_5 are not contiguous. They also occur with a dominant R wave, which means that the R wave has a higher amplitude than the S wave. Now, it turns out that a little bit of T wave inversion can be normal in in leads III, aVR, and V_1, but any sign of T wave inversion in leads V_2 to V_6 is abnormal **(Figure 8.9)**.

SUBENDOCARDIAL INFARCTION

Next, let's look at subendocardial infarction. If the coronary artery remains blocked for around 20 minutes, the subendocardial cells begin to die, which results in necrosis. Just like in subendocardial and transmural ischemia, there's ST depression. Given that there's necrosis, we'd expect there to be leakage of troponin and CK-MB, so this would be an infarction without ST elevation, an NSTEMI, which can again show ST depression and T wave inversion **(Figure 8.10)**.

TRANSMURAL INFARCTION

The final box is for transmural infarction. This occurs when a coronary artery becomes completely blocked for greater than about 20 minutes, which causes transmural necrosis **(Figure 8.11)**. Within minutes, a transmural infarction leads to ECG changes. The most common change is T wave inversions, but there might also be hyperacute T waves, which are large asymmetric T waves that appear in at least two contiguous leads. The classic sign of transmural infarction is ST elevation; when this happens, it's called an ST-elevation myocardial infarction, or STEMI. On ECG, the ST elevation at the J point must be over 1 mm in any two contiguous leads, except V_2 or V_3, where it has to be over 2 mm **(Figure 8.12)**.

ST elevation can also be caused by other conditions, such as coronary artery vasospasm, left ventricular hypertrophy, and pericarditis. For example, a physically fit 20-year-old with a viral illness, who gradually develops chest pain and is found to have ST-elevation on ECG, is more likely to have pericarditis than an ST-elevation myocardial infarction **(Figure 8.13)**.

Transmural infarction can also cause pathologic Q waves to appear on the ECG. Normally, depolarization in the ventricle spreads from the endocardium to the epicardium; most of this wave ends up pointing toward the positive electrode, which means a positive deflection. However, infarcted tissue doesn't conduct electricity, which means that the electrode essentially sees through the infarcted tissue, as if it was a hole, to the *other* ventricular wall. Therefore, the electrode sees the depolarization wave that moves through the healthy wall on the opposite side of the heart. Because those waves are mostly moving away from the positive electrode, you end up with a big, negative pathologic Q wave. So, pathologic Q waves are waves that are longer than .04 seconds, or one small box, and over 2 mm, or two small boxes deep **(Figure 8.14)**.

The location of the transmural infarction can be identified based on the lead that has pathologic Q waves. Septal wall infarctions show changes in leads V_1 and V_2, whereas anterior wall infarctions show changes in leads V_3 and V_4. Anterolateral wall infarctions show up in leads I, V_3 through V_6, and aVL. Small subendocardial infarctions don't cause pathologic Q waves because some of the affected wall still conducts electricity. Also, the aVR lead is oriented in a way that normally produces Q waves, so it's not a reliable lead to look for pathologic Q waves. Finally, pathologic Q waves can also result from things other than transmural infarction, like a left bundle branch block or Wolff-Parkinson-White syndrome **(Figure 8.15)**.

Figure 8.13

ST ELEVATION

* OTHER CAUSES:
  ~ CORONARY ARTERY VASOSPASM
  ~ LEFT VENTRICULAR HYPERTROPHY
  ~ PERICARDITIS

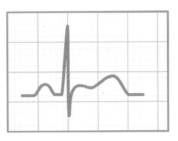

EXAMPLE ~ 20 year old PHYSICALLY FIT PERSON with VIRAL ILLNESS
  ↳ PERICARDITIS ✓
  ↳ STEMI ✗

Figure 8.14

TRANSMURAL INFARCTION

* PATHOLOGIC Q-WAVES

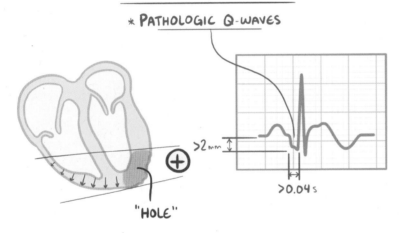

>2 mm

>0.04 s

"HOLE"

Figure 8.15

TRANSMURAL INFARCTION

* PATHOLOGIC Q-WAVES

INFARCT LOCATION	LEAD(S) with PATHOLOGIC QWAVE
SEPTAL WALL	V1, V2
ANTERIOR WALL	V3, V4
ANTEROLATERAL WALL	V3-V6, I, aVL
SUBENDOCARDIAL	NONE

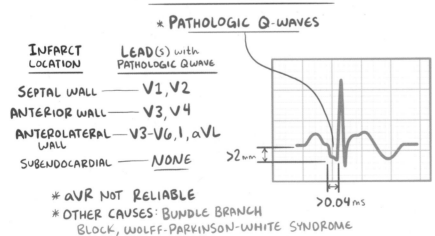

>2 mm

>0.04 ms

* aVR NOT RELIABLE
* OTHER CAUSES: BUNDLE BRANCH BLOCK, WOLFF-PARKINSON-WHITE SYNDROME

Figure 8.16

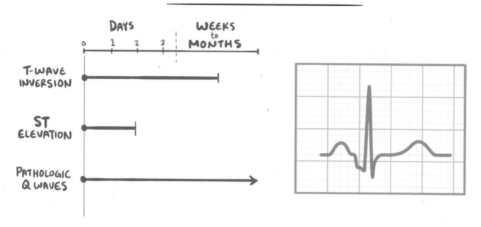

TRANSMURAL INFARCTION

After a transmural myocardial infarction, the ECG gradually begins to look more normal. During the first two days there might be T wave inversion, ST segment elevation, and pathologic Q waves. Around day three, the ST segment is often back at baseline. After a few weeks or months, the T wave inversion may start to improve as well, but pathologic Q waves can linger for much longer. That's why it's always important to compare ECGs to previous ones to look for new changes **(Figure 8.16)**.

SUMMARY

All right, let's quickly recap. Subendocardial ischemia can reflect stable angina, and can cause ST depressions. Transmural ischemia and subendocardial infarction can reflect unstable angina and NSTEMI, and can cause ST depressions and T wave inversions. The two conditions are distinguished from one another by the presence of cardiac enzymes, including CK-MB and troponin. Transmural infarction most often reflects a STEMI, and causes T wave inversions and hyperacute T waves, ST elevation, and pathologic Q waves **(Figure 8.17)**.

Figure 8.17

	ISCHEMIA	INFARCTION
SUBENDOCARDIAL	~ STABLE ANGINA ST DEPRESSIONS	~ UNSTABLE ANGINA ~ NSTEMI ST DEPRESSION T-WAVE INVERSION
TRANSMURAL	~ UNSTABLE ANGINA ~ NSTEMI ST DEPRESSION T-WAVE INVERSION	~ STEMI T-WAVE INVERSIONS HYPERACUTE T-WAVES ST ELEVATION PATHOLOGIC Q WAVES

SOURCES

ELECTROCARDIOGRAPHY BASICS

Dubin, D. (2000). *Dubin's Method for Reading EKG's: Rapid Interpretation of EKG's*. Tampa, FL: COVER Publishing Co. 333-346. Retrieved August 15, 2017, from https://tmedweb.tulane.edu/portal/files/open-access/clinical-diagnosis/ekg_reference_sheets.pdf

Wagner, G. S. & Strauss, D. (2013). *Marriott's Practical Electrocardiography* (12 edition). Philadelphia, PA: Lippincott, Williams & Wilkins.

NORMAL SINUS RHYTHM

Dubin, D. (2000). *Dubin's Method for Reading EKG's: Rapid Interpretation of EKG's*. Tampa, FL: COVER Publishing Co. Retrieved August 15, 2017, from https://tmedweb.tulane.edu/portal/files/open-access/clinical-diagnosis/ekg_reference_sheets.pdf

Yoo, B. (n.d.). Normal sinus rhythm in an EKG. In *Khan Academy Medicine*. Retrieved September 4, 2017, from https://www.khanacademy.org/science/health-and-medicine/circulatory-system-diseases/dysrhythmias-and-tachycardias/v/normal-sinus-rhythm-on-ecg

RATE & RHYTHM

Becker, D. E. (2006). Fundamentals of electrocardiography interpretation. *Anesthesia Progress 53*(2), 53-64. Retrieved September 4, 2017, from https://www.ncbi.nlm.nih.gov/pmc/articles/PMC1614214/

Dubin, D. (2000). *Dubin's Method for Reading EKG's: Rapid Interpretation of EKG's*. Tampa, FL: COVER Publishing Co. Retrieved August 15, 2017, from https://tmedweb.tulane.edu/portal/files/open-access/clinical-diagnosis/ekg_reference_sheets.pdf

AXIS

Ashley, E. A. & Niebauer, J. (2004). Chapter 3: conquering the ECG. *Cardiology Explained* (n.p.). London: Remedica. Retrieved September 1, 2017, from https://www.ncbi.nlm.nih.gov/books/NBK2214/

Dubin, D. (2000). *Dubin's Method for Reading EKG's: Rapid Interpretation of EKG's*.Tampa, FL: COVER Publishing Co. 333-346. Retrieved August 15, 2017, from https://tmedweb.tulane.edu/portal/files/open-access/clinical-diagnosis/ekg_reference_sheets.pdf

Hexaxial reference system (n.d.). In Wikipedia. Retrieved September 1, 2017, from https://en.wikipedia.org/wiki/Hexaxial_reference_system

Karius, D. R. (n.d.). ECG primer: the leads of a 12-lead ECG. In *Kansas City University of Medicine and Biosciences*. Retrieved September 1, 2017, from https://courses.kcumb.edu/physio/ecg%20primer/ecgleads.htm

Thaier, Malcolm S. (2007). *The Only EKG Book You'll Ever Need*. Philadelphia, PA: Lippincott, Williams & Wilkins.

INTERVALS

Abnormalities in the ECG measurements. (n.d.). In *ECG Learning Center, University of Utah*. Retrieved September 1, 2017, from http://ecg.utah.edu/lesson/4

Atrial flutter. (2017). In *MedMovie.com*.Retrieved September 1, 2017, from http://medmovie.com/library_id/4979/topic/cvml_0329a/

Becker, D. E. (2006). Fundamentals of electrocardiography interpretation. *Anesth Prog 53*(2), 53-64.Retrieved September 1, 2017, from https://www.ncbi.nlm.nih.gov/pmc/articles/PMC1614214/

Characteristics of the normal ECG. (n.d.). In *ECG Learning Center, University of Utah*. Retrieved September 1, 2017, from http://ecg.utah.edu/lesson/3

Drug-induced QT interval prolongation and torsades de pointes. (n.d.). In *U.S. Food & Drug Administration*. Retrieved September 1, 2017, from https://www.fda.gov/ohrms/dockets/ac/01/slides/3746s_01_ruskin/sld001.htm

EKG lesson 1. (n.d.). In *Loyola University Stritch School of Medicine*. Retrieved September 1, 2017, from http://www.meddean.luc.edu/lumen/meded/medicine/skills/ekg/les1prnt.htm

EKG lesson 2. (n.d.). In *Loyola University Stritch School of Medicine*. Retrieved September 1, 2017, from http://www.meddean.luc.edu/lumen/meded/medicine/skills/ekg/les2prnt.htm

Goldenberg, I. (2006). QT interval: how to measure it and what is "normal". *J Cardiovasc Electrophysiol*

17(3), 33-336. Retrieved September 1, 2017, from http://www.medscape.com/viewarticle/525633_2

Introduction to ECG rhythm analysis. (n.d.). In *ECG Learning Center, University of Utah*. Retrieved September 1, 2017, from http://ecg.utah.edu/lesson/5-1.

Burns, E. (n.d.). QT interval. In *Life in the Fastlane*. Retrieved September 1, 2017, from https://lifeinthefastlane.com/ecg-library/basics/qt_interval/

QRS TRANSITION

Dubin, D. (2000). *Dubin's Method for Reading EKG's: Rapid Interpretation of EKG's*. Tampa, FL: COVER Publishing Co. Retrieved August 15, 2017, from https://tmedweb.tulane.edu/portal/files/open-access/clinical-diagnosis/ekg_reference_sheets.pdf

Prutkin, J. M. (2016). ECG tutorial: miscellaneous diagnoses. In *UpToDate*. Retrieved September 1, 2017, from https://www.uptodate.com/contents/ecg-tutorial-miscellaneous-diagnoses#H4

Wagner, G. S. & Strauss, D. (2013). *Marriott's Practical Electrocardiography* (12 edition). Philadelphia, PA: Lippincott, Williams & Wilkins.

CARDIAC HYPERTROPHY & ENLARGEMENT

Dubin, D. (2000). *Dubin's Method for Reading EKG's: Rapid Interpretation of EKG's*. Tampa, FL: COVER Publishing Co. Retrieved August 15, 2017, from https://tmedweb.tulane.edu/portal/files/open-access/clinical-diagnosis/ekg_reference_sheets.pdf

Wagner, G. S. & Strauss, D. (2013). *Marriott's Practical Electrocardiography* (12 edition). Philadelphia, PA: Lippincott, Williams & Wilkins.

CARDIAC INFARCTION & ISCHEMIA

Burns, E. (n.d.). Myocardial ischaemia. In *Life in the Fastlane*. Retrieved September 1, 2017, from https://lifeinthefastlane.com/ecg-library/myocardial-ischaemia/

Conti, C. Richard. (2013). *The Netter Collection of Medical Illustrations - Cardiovascular System E-Book*. Amsterdam: Elsevier Health Sciences.

Dubin, D. (2000). *Dubin's Method for Reading EKG's: Rapid Interpretation of EKG's*. Tampa, FL: COVER

Publishing Co. Retrieved August 15, 2017, from https://tmedweb.tulane.edu/portal/files/open-access/clinical-diagnosis/ekg_reference_sheets.pdf

Goldberger, A. L. & Prutkin, J. M. (2016). Electrocardiogram in the diagnosis of myocardial ischemia and infarction. In *UpToDate*. Retrieved September 1, 2017, from https://www.uptodate.com/contents/electrocardiogram-in-the-diagnosis-of-myocardial-ischemia-and-infarction

Nable, Jose Victor, and William Brady. (2009). The evolution of electrocardiographic changes in ST-segment elevation myocardial infarction. *The American Journal of Emergency Medicine* 27(6), 734–46. Retrieved September 1, 2017, from 10.1016/j.ajem.2008.05.025

Thygesen, Kristian, Joseph S. Alpert, Allan S. Jaffe, Maarten L. Simoons, Bernard R. Chaitman, and Harvey D. White. (2012). Third universal definition of myocardial infarction. *Circulation 126*(16), 2020–35. Retrieved September 1, 2017, from https://www.ncbi.nlm.nih.gov/pubmed/22923432

Wagner, G. S. & Strauss, D. (2013). *Marriott's Practical Electrocardiography* (12 edition). Philadelphia, PA: Lippincott, Williams & Wilkins.

INDEX

Numbers in red indicate the term is defined on those pages.

T

U

V

W